Pharmacy Management Software

for Pharmacy Technicians

A WORKTEXT

DAA Enterprises, Inc.

BROOKLINE, MASSACHUSETTS

WRITTEN BY

Karen Davis, AAHCA, CPhT

ALLIED HEALTH PROGRAM SPECIALIST
VIRGINIA COLLEGES
BIRMINGHAM, ALABAMA

SECOND EDITION

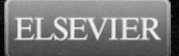

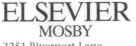
MOSBY

3251 Riverport Lane
St. Louis, Missouri 63043

PHARMACY MANAGEMENT SOFTWARE   ISBN: 978-0-323-07554-1
FOR PHARMACY TECHNICIANS: A WORKTEXT
SECOND EDITION

Notice

Neither the Publisher nor the Author assumes any responsibility for any loss or injury and/or damage to persons or property arising out of or related to any use of the material contained in this book. It is the responsibility of the treating practitioner, relying on independent expertise and knowledge of the patient, to determine the best treatment and method of application for the patient.

The Publisher

International Standard Book Number: 978-0-323-07554-1

Vice President and Publisher: Andrew Allen
Senior Acquisitions Editor: Jennifer Janson
Developmental Editor: Kelly Brinkman
Compositor: GraphCom Corporation
Designer: Paula Catalano

Printed in the United States of America
Last digit is the print number: 9 8 7 6 5 4 3 2 1

Preface

Welcome to the exciting world of Pharmacy Technology! You have started on a journey into one of today's fastest-growing fields in health care. Whether you will end up working in an institutional pharmacy, a community pharmacy, one of the large pharmacy chain stores, or another location, the skills that you will gain from *Pharmacy Management Software for Pharmacy Technicians* will help prepare you well for your new career.

Pharmacy technicians are increasingly called on to perform duties traditionally fulfilled by pharmacists. This is because of new federal regulations that now require pharmacists to spend more time with patients providing patient education. Because of the nature of the pharmacy technician's work, hands-on training is critically important in educational programs. This software package is designed to provide hands-on training and help you master the information and skills necessary to be a successful pharmacy technician. The various activities will challenge your knowledge, help further reinforce key concepts, and allow you to gauge your understanding of the subject matter studied in your pharmacy technician program.

Pharmacy Management Software for Pharmacy Technicians is a reliable and an understandable resource written specifically for the pharmacy technician student. The worktext is divided into four sections—Community Pharmacy Practice, Institutional Pharmacy Practice, Reports, and Assessment. Each section guides you through the various tasks that pharmacy technicians are expected to be able to perform in a pharmacy setting.

Contents

Introduction

Installation

1   Close all programs.

2   Insert the DVD labeled *Pharmacy Management Software for Pharmacy Technicians* into your DVD-ROM drive. If Auto run is enabled on your system, this dialog box will be displayed. If Auto run is not enabled:

    a From the **START** menu, select **RUN**.

    b Type **D:\SETUP** (substitute the appropriate letter of your DVD-ROM drive for D).

    c Press **ENTER** or click on the **INSTALL** button to start installation.

3   The Installation Wizard will start to guide the rest of the setup. Click **NEXT** to view the End User License Agreement screen. Read the End User License Agreement carefully.

4   Select **I ACCEPT** and click **NEXT**.

5   Select the destination folder. By default, the software is installed in C:\Program Files\.

    Another dialog box prompts you for installation type. Select **STANDALONE** or **SERVER INSTALLATION**.

6   A final confirmation dialog box shows you all setup settings. Click **NEXT** to start copying the software from the DVD to your computer. After all files have copied, click **FINISH**. You may need to restart your computer to access the software after installation.

Navigating Visual SuperScript: The Basics

Understanding the basics of software navigation is essential to your success in this course. If you are already familiar with Microsoft Windows applications, such as Word or Excel, you already have the necessary basic navigation knowledge. However, even if you are new to using a computer, you should be able to navigate the software after learning a few key concepts.

- The first screen that you will see after installing the software is the main menu.

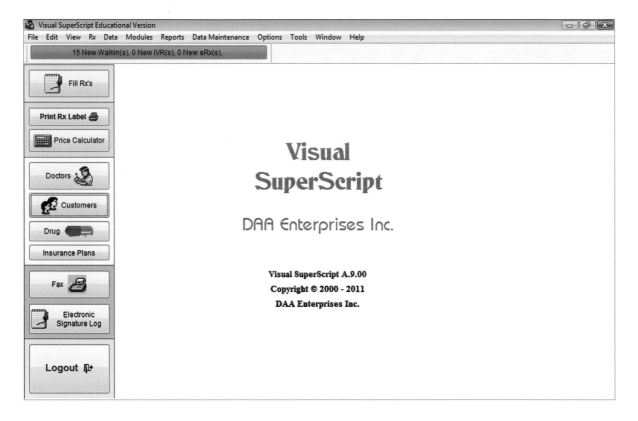

- When you click on a menu choice that appears across the top of the main menu, you will see a drop-down list. Each menu choice on that drop-down list appears with one letter underlined. That letter represents a "hot key" for that choice. Each item on the menu may be selected by pressing the Alt key and the corresponding hot key at the same time. For example, an Activity Summary may be selected from the **REPORTS/ADMIN REPORTS** menu by pressing on the A key. Of course, you may also select any menu option by moving the mouse pointer to it and clicking on it.

Reports	Data Maintenance	Options	Tools	Window	Help

Report Manager...

Admin Reports ▸	Activity Summary
	Profit Summary
Mailing Labels ▸	Detail Summary
Daily Prescription Log ▸	Reversed Rx List
	Sales tax Report
Doctor Reports ▸	Rx Percentage Report
Customer Reports ▸	Hourly Workload Report
Drug Reports ▸	Rx's Below AWP Cost
Third Party Reports ▸	Rx's Revenue percentage by state
Refill Reminders ▸	
Delivery Reports ▸	
Transferred Rx's List	
Price Exception Report	
Warning Labels	

Note: Unless indicated otherwise, "Clicking the mouse" or "Clicking on it" means clicking the left mouse button once. On certain occasions you will need to click the left button twice quickly. This is called "double clicking." Certain features of the program are accessed through menus that are displayed by clicking the right mouse button once. This is called "right clicking."

Objects, Icons, and Controls

You will interact with the software by using the various objects that appear in each dialog box. Some objects appear as buttons with small pictures on them. These will be referred to as icons. Other objects appear as check boxes, simple data entry areas referred to as text boxes or fields, and drop-down lists and combo boxes.

In most dialog boxes, data can be entered a multiple of ways. Several text boxes and a few check boxes may be offered. The blinking cursor will provide a visual cue as to where you are in the form. To move from one space on a form to another, pressing the Tab key is best.

Text boxes

Text boxes are the most common objects that you will encounter. They are used to type in data or display numbers, such as names, DEA numbers, and dates. Example of text boxes are the **Rx No.**, **Disp Date**, and **RPh Initials** boxes on the Rx Processing form.

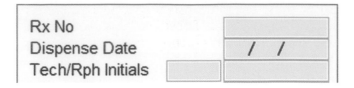

Some text boxes may be "read-only," meaning they can only display information. Information cannot be added or changed in read-only text boxes.

List boxes

List boxes are used when only certain responses can be used for a specific part of a form. Each list box has a downward small arrow next to it. You can see what choices you have for a text box by clicking on the downward arrow and then clicking on the response of your choice. For example, when entering how a customer is going to pay for prescriptions, the user clicks on the arrow to the right of the pay type text box and then selects either private or insurance from the drop-down list.

```
ABSTON, KINLEY B
03/23/1926      Q Code  KA032326
INSURANCE                        ▼
INSURANCE                        ▼
PRIVATE
```

Combo boxes

Combo boxes are very similar to list boxes; however, there are some differences. Visually, a combo box has a small icon next to it like a drop-down list, except the arrow has a line below it. The most important difference, however, is that the content in a combo box can be changed, unlike the content from a drop-down list. Combo boxes allow you to add, change, or remove information.

Icons

Icons, or buttons with pictures on them, appear throughout the software. However, you will mostly see icons on the **FILE NAVIGATION TOOLBAR** that appears at the top of your screen.

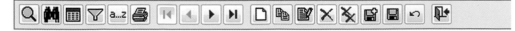

All of these buttons appear whenever a form that is designed for data entry is being used. These buttons are referred to as the navigation tools, and the bar on which they appear is called the toolbar.

Each button has a picture that provides a clue about its function. A slightly more detailed explanation of the button's purpose may be obtained by moving the mouse pointer to a button and holding it there for several seconds. A small description of the button will appear.

The toolbar icons and corresponding purpose are as follows:

FIND button

This button is used to help find records.

LOCATE button

This button is used to locate records that meet certain criteria, such as families that live in a certain zip code.

LIST button

This button enables you to display the records in a file as a list.

FILTER button

The filter button allows you to set filters so that only certain subsets of records are displayed. The filter function is similar to the locate function.

SORT button

The sort button allows you to select the order in which records are displayed.

PRINT button

This button allowed you to print the record(s) that you are currently viewing.

NEXT button

This button moves you to the next record in a table.

LAST button

This button moves you to the last record in a table.

NEW button

Clicking this button displays a blank form to begin adding a new record.

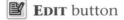 **COPY** button

Clicking this button makes a copy of the current record and displays it for editing. This feature is handy when much of the information on a newly created record can be carried over from another record.

EDIT button

Clicking this button allows you to make changes to a record.

DELETE button

Clicking this button deletes the current record.

GROUP DELETE button

This button allows a group of records that meet a certain criteria to be deleted.

MORE button

This button saves the current record and displays a blank form for adding a new record.

SAVE button

This button saves the current record.

CANCEL button

This button cancels all changes made to the current record since the last time the record was saved.

CLOSE button

This button closes the form.

COMMUNITY PHARMACY PRACTICE

LAB 1

Adding a Physician or Prescriber to the Database

LAB OBJECTIVES

In this lab, you will:

- Learn to add a physician or prescriber to the database.

STUDENT DIRECTIONS

Estimated completion time: 30 minutes

1. Read through the steps in the lab before performing the lab exercise.
2. After reading through the lab, perform the required steps to enter provider information.
3. Complete the exercise at the end of the lab.

R̟x

Dr. Larry Peterson
11321 9th Street
Learning, IA 50115
Office: (717) 330-1990, ext. 109
Fax: (717) 330-1991

Patient Name: _____

Date: _____

Address: _____

     Refill: _____
     Rx:

Product Selection Permitted   Dispense As Written

DEA: BP1234892

Address: _____

State License: 073223

Steps to Add a Physician or Prescriber to the Database

1   Access the main screen of Visual SuperScript.

2   Click on the **DOCTORS** button located on the left side of the screen. A dialog box entitled *Doctors* will pop up.

3   Click on the **FIND** 🔍 icon located on the top left of the toolbar. A dialog box entitled *Doctor Lookup* will pop up.

4   Enter the first three letters of the prescriber's last name in the **NAME** field.

          Enter *PET* for Dr. Larry Peterson.

5   If the doctor is not found in the list, click **ADD**. The form is now ready for you to enter the prescriber information.

> **LAB TIP:** You may click **ENTER** after typing in the first three letters of the doctor's name. If the prescriber is not in the database, the *Add Doctor* box will appear. Click **YES, MANUALLY**, to add the new prescriber.

6   The **NAME** is a required field. Enter the prescriber name starting with the last name, followed by a comma, one space, and then the first name.

Enter *Peterson, Larry* for Dr. Larry Peterson.

7   The **CONTACT** field should contain the name of the person you usually talk to when you call the doctor's office for refill authorization.

Enter *Brandon* as the contact.

8   Enter the prescriber's **ADDRESS**.

Enter *11321 9th Street, Learning, IA 50115* as the address.

The city and zip code of the prescriber are not in the database. A pop-up table entitled *Zip* appears after entering the zip code.

9   Scroll through the *Zip* pop-up table to ensure that the desired zip code and city information are not in the database. Then click **CANCEL** at the bottom of the box. The *Zip* pop-up table will close out and the *Doctors* form will again be active.

10 To add the city and zip code to the database, right click the **ZIP CODE** data entry field. A drop-down menu appears.

   a Choose **ADD NEW** from the drop-down menu. A pop-up dialog box appears entitled *Zip Codes*.

   b Enter the prescriber zip code, city, and state abbreviation.

   c Click on the **SAVE** 🖫 icon located at the top right of the dialog box toolbar.

   d Click on the **CLOSE** 🗗 icon located at the top right of the toolbar.

11 Press the **TAB** key to navigate through the address fields. The zip code information has now been added to the database. Verify that the correct zip code information has been added by clicking on the **COMBO-BOX ARROW** located to the right of the zip code data entry field.

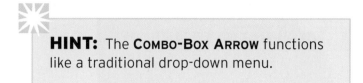

HINT: The **COMBO-BOX ARROW** functions like a traditional drop-down menu.

Note: If the zip code is in the database, the city and state fields will populate automatically.

12 Enter the prescriber's **PHONE** information.

Enter *717/330-1990 extension 109* as the office phone.
Enter *717/330-1991* as the fax number.

13 Enter the prescriber's initials in the **QUICK CODES** field.

14 Enter *BP1234892* as the **DEA** number.

15 Enter *073223* as the **STATE LICENSE** number.

16 Enter *073223* as the prescriber's **MEDICARD** number.

17 Keep the **COVERED BY MEDICAID** check box checked if the prescriber is authorized to write prescriptions for Medicaid-supported patients.

Dr. Peterson is authorized to write prescriptions for Medicaid-supported patients.

18 Click on the **ARROW** to the right of the **HOSPITAL** field.

Select *CITY HOSPITAL.*

19 Click on the **ARROW** to the right of the **STATUS** field.

Select ACTIVE from the drop-down list to indicate that the prescriber is in active practicing status.

20 Click on the **SAVE** 💾 icon located at the top right of the dialog box toolbar.

21   Print the screen by using the **PRINTSCRN** option on your keyboard. Press the **PRINTSCRN** key, open a blank Word document, **RIGHT CLICK** the blank Word document, and then select **PASTE**.

22   Check with your instructor on the preferred method for submitting your work.

23   Click the **CLOSE** [icon] icon located at the top right of the dialog box toolbar.

Exercise

Practice using the software data entry skills by entering the following prescriber information. Follow step 21 for each prescriber who is added to the database. Submit work when completed.

Note: A message box will appear indicating that the DEA number is invalid. Click **No** and continue entering the prescriber's information.

Prescriber Information

Dr. Catelynn Judith
9608 Barroll Lane, Suite 333
Kensington, MD 20895
Phone: 301-962-3140
Fax: 301-962-3144
DEA: AJ1256948-012
State License/Medicaid: 077332
Contact: Jen

Dr. Emma Francis
2208 Colonial Acres Court, Suite 444
Herndon, VA 20170
Phone: 703-430-3814
Fax: 703-430-3813
DEA: BF2368521
State License/Medicaid: 023569
Contact: Office Secretary

Dr. Markus Wayne
1812 Lincoln Highway, #52
Reston, VA 20190
Phone: 703-829-1100
Fax: 703-829-1111
DEA: AW7899562-134
State License/Medicaid: 096587
Contact: Judy

Dr. Jennifer Suz
1800 Lincoln Highway
Reston, VA 20194-1215
Phone: 703-829-1000
Fax: 703-829-1100
DEA: AS5478547
State License/Medicaid: 056921
Contact: Joe

Dr. Jacob Field
7500 Evans Street
Sterling, VA 20197
Phone: 703-571-2344
Fax: 703-571-2345
DEA: BF8527414
State License/Medicaid: 098632
Contact: Assistant—Ralph

Dr. Lucille Moore
7500 Evans Street
Pittsburgh, PA 15218
Phone: 412-571-2300
Fax: 412-571-2301
DEA: AM5698523
State License/Medicaid: 000234
Contact: none

Dr. Tom Pane
5121 Brightwood Road, #110
Bethel Park, PA 15102
Phone: 412-835-4700
Fax: 412-835-4701
DEA: AP6985213
State License/Medicaid: 045698
Contact: Brenda

Dr. D. Kraft
11818 "F" Street
Omaha, NE 68137
Phone: 402-899-9911
Fax: 402-891-9912
DEA: AK2566326
State License/Medicaid: 023695
Contact: Brecken

Dr. I. Audubon
109 Eastside Drive
Omaha, NE 68137
Phone: 402-891-5521
Fax: 402-891-5522
DEA: AA7856412
State License/Medicaid: 030256
Contact: Office Nurse

Prescriber Name:
Prescriber Address:
Phone:
Fax:
DEA:
State License/Medicaid:
Contact:

HINT: When adding a group of prescribers at the same time, click the **MORE** icon located on the top right of the dialog box toolbar. Use the **MORE** icon in place of the **SAVE** icon.

Adding a New Patient to the Database

LAB OBJECTIVES

In this lab, you will:

- Learn how to add a new patient to the pharmacy software database.

STUDENT DIRECTIONS

Estimated completion time: 30 minutes

1. Read through the steps in the lab before performing the lab exercise.
2. After reading through the lab, perform the required steps to enter patient information.
3. Complete the exercise at the end of the lab.

Steps to Add a New Patient to the Database

1   Access the main screen of Visual SuperScript.

2   Click on the **CUSTOMERS** button located on the left side of the screen. A dialog box entitled *Customers* will pop up.

3   Click on the **FIND** 🔍 icon located on the dialog box toolbar. A dialog box entitled *Customer Lookup* pops up.

4   Search the database to be certain the patient is not already entered.

Type *She* and scroll through to check for patient Mary Shedlock.

5   Click on **ADD** at the bottom of the dialog screen to begin entering the patient. The *Customers* dialog box opens, the form is now ready to enter new patient information.

> **LAB TIP:** You may click **ENTER** after typing in the first three letters of the patient's name. If the patient is not in the database, click **YES** when you are asked "Add Customer?"

6   Type the patient's name in the **NAME** field.

Enter *Shedlock, Mary E.* as the patient name.

Note: The **NAME** is a required field and allows up to 30 characters. The recommended format is last name followed by a comma, a single space, first name, a single space, middle initial or middle name, if known.

> **HINT:** To facilitate searching your database, following the recommended format for entering names is very important. **Last names are entered first.** Example: Johnson, Linda P.

7   Enter Mary's date of birth in the **BIRTHDATE** field.

Enter *03/03/1960.*

> **HINT:** The format for entering birth-dates into the database is mm/dd/yyyy. Example: 06/07/1964 (Do not enter as 6/7/1964.)

8   Enter the patient's initials into the **Q CODES** field.

Enter *MS* for patient's initials.

> **HINT: Q CODES** (Quick Codes) allow you to expedite the search for customers when filling prescriptions.

9   Click on the **ARROW** located to the right of the **PAY TYPE** data entry field. Select appropriate **PAY TYPE**.

Select *Private.*

Note: PAY TYPE determines how prescriptions filled for this patient are priced and who is expected to pay for them. Two **PAY TYPES** are permissible: *Private* and *Insurance.*

10   Click on the **ARROW** located to the right of the **GENDER** data entry field.

Select appropriate gender as *Female.*

11   Tab to the **FAMILY** field. A pop-up dialog box asking, "Is customer also head of family?" will come up. Click **No**. When you are prompted to add, click **YES**, and enter *Matthew Shedlock* as the family head.

Note: FAMILY is a required field. Customers are grouped into families, with each family having one individual designated as the **FAMILY HEAD**. Each customer is linked to the family database by reference to the **FAMILY HEAD**.

> **HINT:** The abbreviation *HOH* stands for *Head of Household,* which indicates the family head.

12   Enter the address and phone number information in the *Families* screen. Once the following information is entered, **SAVE** 💾 and **CLOSE** out of *Families*.

Enter *1386 Quincy Lane, Allston, MA 02134. 703-464-0100*

13   Tab to the **NOTES** field.

Enter notes: *Patient is hard of hearing in left ear.*

Note: You can enter whatever information you want to store about the patient in the **NOTES** field. The information will appear on the *Prescription Processing* screen as a reminder when filling a prescription for this patient.

14   Enter the **DRIVER'S LICENSE** and **SOCIAL SECURITY** numbers in their respective fields.

DL: *057915228*
SS#: *111-22-2333*

15   Tab to the **RX ELIGIBILITY** and the **LOCATION CODE** fields.

Enter *Dependent Parent* and *Home* where prompted.

16   Tab to the **CHILDPROOF OPTION** field. By default, this box will be **CP** for every customer that is added to the database.

Leave the default CP setting for Mary.

Note: The law requires the use of a child-proof lid unless specified otherwise. If a customer desires easy-open lids, use the drop-down menu and indicate this here.

17   Tab to the **NO OF LABELS** field. Indicate a *1* in this field unless the patient requests two labels at the time the prescription for this patient is filled.

Mary only needs one label right now.

18   Click on the **ALLERGIES** tab bottom half of the *Customers* form

19   Click on the **NEW** 🗋 icon located on the bottom right of the *Customers* form. An *Allergen Lookup* table pops up.

20   Key in the first two letters of the allergy in the **ALLERGY** data entry field. Use the scroll bar to select the appropriate allergy. Select the appropriate allergy by clicking on the allergy and then click **OK**.

Key in *MOR*. Select *morphine*. Click *OK*.

21   Click on the **OTHER DRUGS** tab.

22   Click on the **NEW** 🗋 icon located on the bottom right of the *Customers* form. Press the **ENTER** key to access a list of drugs. A *Drug Name Lookup* table pops up.

Note: The **OTHER DRUGS** grid contains information about other drugs that the patient is currently taking. These prescription drugs may have been purchased from a different pharmacy, or they may be over-the-counter (OTC) drugs. For each such drug, a start date and estimated days of supply may also be entered. The purpose of recording this information is to check for possible drug interactions and duplicate ingredients and therapy.

23   Type the name of the drug in the **NAME** dialog box to look up the drug. Click on the desired drug to select it. Click on **OK**.

Mary Shedlock began taking Vitamin E 400 softgel qd in 12/2006.

24   Click on the **DISEASE PROFILE** tab.

25   Click on the **NEW** 🗋 icon located on the bottom right of the *Customers* form. A red bar appears across the *Disease Profile* table. Click inside the *Disease Profile* to turn blue (which indicates information can be entered).

Note: The **DISEASE PROFILE** grid contains a list of diseases for which the customer has been diagnosed. The information contained in this grid is used to check for drug-disease contraindications each time a prescription is filled for the patient.

26   A *Disease Lookup* table pops up entitled **CFDBDX**. Look up the disease by typing the first few letters of the name of the disease. Click on the desired disease to select it. Click on **OK**.

Enter *diabetes mellitus–noninsulin-dependent* for the disease.

27   Click on the **SAVE** 🖫 icon located at the top right of the toolbar in the *Customers* dialog box.

Customers (1)

Customer	Workers Comp Information	InPatient Info	Miscellaneous

Name SHEDLOCK, MARY E	Driver License ▾ 057915228
Birthdate 03/03/1960 Q Code MS	Social Security # 111-22-3333
Pay Type PRIVATE ▾	Rx Eligibility Dependent Parent ▾
Gender FEMALE ▾	Location Code Home ▾
Family SHEDLOCK, MATTHEW	Nursing Home ⬇
Notes patient is hard of hearing in left ear. ▲	ChildProof Option CP ⬇
	No Of Labels 1
Highlight During Rx Processing ☐ ▼	View Signatures MediCare Elig. Check

Per Diem Information

Diet Orders	Lab Orders	Rehab Orders	Restorative Nursing Orders	Treatment Orders	Ancillary Orders	Admission
Insurance Plans		Allergies	Other Drugs	Disease Profile		ID Cards

Disease	▲
DIABETES MELL./NON-INS. DEPEND	
	▼

◀   ▶

---

28   Print the screen by using the **PRINTSCRN** option on your keyboard: Press the **PRINTSCRN** key, open a blank Word document, **RIGHT CLICK** the blank Word document, and then select **PASTE**.

29   Click the **CLOSE** 🔳 icon located at the top right of the toolbar.

Exercise

Enter the following customers into the database using the information provided. Refer back to Lab 1 if any zip codes are not entered into the database.

Patient and HOH: Ray Ruhl
DOB: 2/21/57
SSN: 472-97-4562
Allergies: penicillin (PCN)
170 Laurel Way
Herndon, VA 20170
Home phone: 703-481-5200
DL: 548492721
Pay type: Private
Requests easy-open caps
No known allergies
Other medications: albuterol inhaler, Singulair 10 mg
Disease state: asthma, diagnosis of

Patient and HOH: Robert Gamble
DOB: 3/15/57
SSN: 423-11-3333
Allergies: PCN
1447 Woodbrook Court
Reston, VA 20194-1215
Home phone: 703-787-9000
Pay type: Private
Hospice patient
Requests easy-open lids
Disease state: cancer
Other medications: Pain medications

Patient: Julie Douglas
HOH: Doug Douglas (same address as Julie)
DOB: 8/14/77
Allergies: codeine
Not pregnant
SSN: 333-56-9887
12124 Walnut Branch Road
Audubon, IA 50025
Home phone: 571-203-0000
Notes: Deliver prescriptions to home address before 5:00 PM

Patient: Katherine Cald
HOH: Timothy Cald
DOB: 3/20/57
DL# I4569821
Allergies: cephalosporins
Insurance plan: Anthem
11200 Longwood Grove
Elk Horn, IA 51531
Home phone: 703-464-1700

Patient and HOH: Annette Mang
DOB: 1/21/57
SSN: 362-89-5663
Allergies: morphine
1490 Autumn Ridge Court
Reston, VA 20194-1215
Home phone: 703-834-0500
Other medications: alprazolam 1 mg, Seroquel 25 mg
Wants duplicate labels

Patient and HOH: Dana Walks
DOB: 4/21/57
Allergies: PCN
1206 Weatherstone Court
Ralston, NE 68128
Home phone: 703-430-6300
Requests easy-open caps
Notes: Has not signed HIPAA form
Other medications: Skelaxin 400 mg PRN, spironolactone 100 mg

Patient and HOH: Martin Marin
DOB: 5/17/50
Allergies: no known allergies (NKA)
11324 Olde Tiverton Circle
Ralston, NE 68128
Home phone: 703-437-5000
Other medications: Aldactone 100 mg, Serevent Inhaler
Would like two labels
Would like easy-open caps
Work-related injury
Contact at work: Steve Thomas—Manager
Bonds, Inc., 309 Third Street, Fister, NE 68110
Work phone: 402-698-2356

> **LAB TIPS:** Use the vertical scroll bar located on the right side of the pop-up dialog box to view customer information. To facilitate searching your database, following the correct naming procedures is very important.

Making a Change to the Patient Profile or Prescriber Information

LAB OBJECTIVES

In this lab, you will:

- Learn how to update patient profiles.
- Learn how to edit prescriber information.

STUDENT DIRECTIONS

Estimated completion time: 20 minutes

1. Read through the steps in the lab before performing the lab exercise.
2. After reading through the lab, perform the required steps to edit or add information.
3. Complete the exercise at the end of the lab.

Steps to Change the Patient Profile or Prescriber Information

1   Access the main screen of Visual SuperScript.

2   Click on the **CUSTOMERS** button located on the left side of the screen. A dialog box entitled *Customers* will pop up.

3   Click on the **FIND** 🔍 icon , which is located on the top left of the *Customers* dialog box toolbar.

4   A dialog box entitled *Customer Lookup* pops up. Enter the first letter of the customer's last name into the **NAME** data entry field. Click on the patient name for whom information will be updated.

Find *John M. Smith.*

5   The selected customer name is highlighted in blue. Click on the **EDIT** icon located at the bottom of the *Customer Lookup* dialog box. A dialog box entitled *Customers* pops up.

6   Click on the **EDIT** 📝 icon located in the middle of the *Customers* toolbar at the top of the dialog box.

7   Tab to the desired data entry field, and key in the appropriate changes.

Change John M. Smith's DOB to *02/22/1947.*

8   Click on the **SAVE** 💾 icon located on the toolbar at the top right of the *Customers* dialog box. A pop-up box will indicate that allergies have not been entered for the customer. Click **No** to indicate that no known allergies exist for this customer. The updated information will then be saved.

9   Click on the **CLOSE** 📲 icon located on the toolbar at the top right of the *Customers* dialog box. The edited information has now been added to the database.

10 Make note of the updated information in the *Customer Lookup* dialog box. Click on **OK** at the bottom of the *Customer Lookup* dialog box.

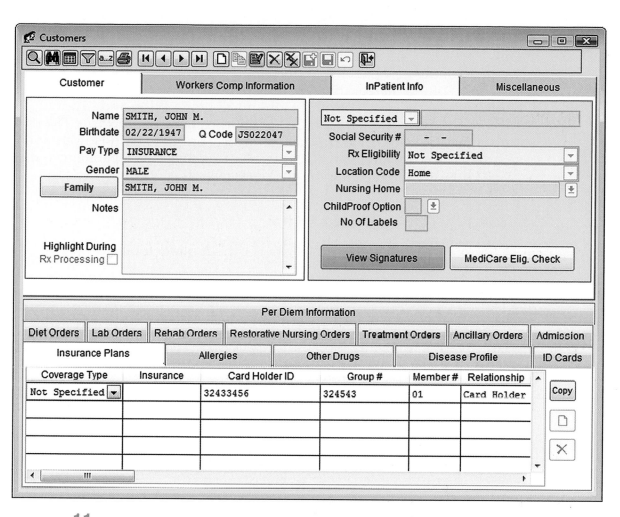

11   Print the screen by using the **PrintScrn** option on your keyboard: Press the **PrintScrn** key, open a blank Word document, **Right Click** the blank Word document, and then select **Paste**.

Exercise

Practice using the software data entry skills by entering the following patient information. Submit work when completed.

Change the following patient information:

- Jada Sanchez's birthday is 08/30/1996.
- Margaret Pena's is the HOH, and her home phone number is 555-639-5489.

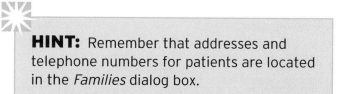

HINT: Remember that addresses and telephone numbers for patients are located in the *Families* dialog box.

Quick Challenge

When adding new patients to the database, it may be necessary, on occasion, to merge customer information. To merge customer information means that you are joining all prescription and history records of one customer with that of another. For example, Don Flowers may have been added to the database twice; once as Dawn Flowers and another time as Don Flowers. Rather than keeping two separate records for one customer, merging the customer records is necessary.

Steps to Merge Customer Records

1 Click on **DATA MAINTENANCE** from the main menu toolbar.

2 Click on **MERGE CUSTOMER RECORDS**.

3 Key in John Smith with John M. Smith in the *Merge Customer Records* dialog box and click **OK**.

> **LAB TIP:** Remember to search for each customer using the last name first.

4 Click **YES** after checking the names in the dialog box to be merged.

Confirmation   ☒

? All prescriptions and history records of

SMITH, JOHN

will be merged with those of

SMITH, JOHN M.

and the former's record will be deleted.

[Yes]   [No]

---

5 The customer records of John Smith with John M. Smith are now merged.

> **Note:** The active data entry field will be highlighted. Delete the existing information before adding the new information.

Steps to Edit a Prescriber Form

1 Access the main screen of Visual SuperScript.

2 Click on the **DOCTORS** button located on the left side of the screen. A dialog box entitled *Doctors* will pop up.

3 Click on the **FIND** 🔍 icon located on the toolbar at the top of the dialog box. The *Find* dialog box appears.

4 The *Find* dialog box offers several choices for locating the prescriber's records. Key in the prescriber's last name in the **NAME** data entry field. Click **OK** at the bottom of the dialog box.

Key in *Dr. Robert Bosworth.*

5 Click on the **EDIT** 📝 icon located on the toolbar at the top of the form. The form is now ready for you to edit the prescriber information.

6 Tab through the form to reach the desired data entry field. Make appropriate changes to the form.

Enter the office phone 2 extension of *104.*

7 Click on the **SAVE** 💾 icon located at the top right of the toolbar.

8 Print the screen by using the **PRINTSCRN** option on your keyboard: Hit the **PRINTSCRN** key, open a blank Word document, **RIGHT CLICK** the blank Word document, and then select **PASTE**.

Exercise

Scenario

Dr. Karen Davis is a prescribing physician in your area. She has recently married and changed her last name to a hyphenated name: Dr. Karen Davis-Bendfeldt. The managing pharmacist has asked you to update Dr. Davis-Bendfeldt's records.

Task

Following the steps from the *Editing a Prescriber Form* exercise, edit Dr. Karen Davis-Bendfeldt's information. Print or save the form, and submit it for verification.

Enter the first letter of the prescriber's last name into the **NAME** data entry field. Click **OK** at the bottom of the dialog box. A dialog box entitled *List* pops up. Scroll through the table in the *List* dialog box, and select the desired prescriber by clicking on the prescriber's name. Click **OK** located at the bottom of the *List* dialog box.

Note: Deleting the existing information before adding the new information is not necessary. Simply key the new information into the highlighted data entry field.

Adding Insurance Plans to the Database

LAB OBJECTIVES

In this lab, you will:

- Learn how to add a new insurance plan to the database.
- Key information regarding insurance billing procedures.

STUDENT DIRECTIONS

Estimated completion time: 45 minutes

1. Read through the steps in the lab before performing the lab exercise.
2. After reading through the lab, perform the required steps listed in the lab.
3. Answer the questions at the end of the lab.
4. Complete the exercise at the end of the lab.

Pre Lab Information

The insurance plan name could be the same name as the insurance company. However, each insurance company generally offers different plans. Not only do these plans have different restrictions and different copay requirements, but they may also need to be submitted with different biller identification numbers (BINs) and/or PROCESSOR CONTROL numbers. Therefore *it is best to avoid associating plan names with insurance company names.*

Similarly, there are Pharmacy Benefits Managers, such as ARGUS and Diversified Pharmacy Services (DPS), who process claims on behalf of large numbers of insurance companies. It is best to avoid associating plan names with the names of these processors either.

Most often, each insurance plan that requires a unique combination of BIN and PROCESSOR CONTROL numbers should have a separate name and a separate record.

Steps to Add Insurance Plans to the Database

1 Access the main screen of Visual SuperScript.

2 Click on the **INSURANCE PLANS** button located on the left side of the screen. A dialog box appears entitled *Insurance Plans*.

> **Note:** The *Insurance Plans* form is used to maintain a database of insurance plans to which your customers subscribe. The *Insurance Plans* form contains three tabs. Be sure the **INSURANCE PLAN DATA** tab is open when following the steps.

3 Click on the **NEW** ▯ icon located on the toolbar at the top of the *Insurance Plans* dialog box. The form is ready for data entry.

4 Enter the name of the insurance plan in the **PLAN NAME** data entry field.

Enter *Medco* as the plan name.

5 Tab to the **COMPANY** data entry field. Type in the first three letters of the company name and hit **ENTER**. A list will then pop up in which you can select the company name.

Choose *United Healthcare* as the company name, and click OK.

6 Tab to the next data entry field underneath *Company Phone*. This field is used to identify the pharmacy to the insurance company for billing purposes. Click on the **ARROW** located to the right of the data entry field. Scroll through the pick list, and select the desired **IDENTIFICATION QUALIFIER** by clicking on the name.

Choose *NCPDP Provider ID* as the identification qualifier.

7 Tab to the next unnamed data entry field. Enter the pharmacy identification (ID) number in the next data entry field.

Enter *6503829* as the pharmacy ID.

> **Note:** In most cases, the unique pharmacy identification number is the National Association Board of Pharmacy (NABP) number.

8 Tab to the **BILLING METHOD** data entry field. Click on the **ARROW** located to the right of the **BILLING METHOD** data entry field. Choose the desired **BILLING METHOD** by clicking on the pick list name.

Choose *electronic billing* as the billing method.

9   Tab to the **Max Days for Refills** data entry field.

Note: This field specifies the period during which prescriptions must be refilled to be eligible for reimbursement under this plan.

Enter *365* as the Max Days for Refills.

10   Tab to the **Max Refills** data entry field.

Enter *6* as the Max Refills.

Note: This field represents the number of times the insurance company will pay on a given prescription to be refilled. A value of zero (0) implies that refills are not allowed.

11   Tab to the **Max Days Supply** data entry field.

Note: This field represents a payer-imposed limit, if any, on the amount of a medication that may be dispensed at a time.

Enter *32* as the Max Days Supply.

12   Check the **Add Sales Tax** check box if your state imposes a sales tax on medicines. The sales tax will then be billed to the insurance company.

13   The **Dis Gen Unless DAW** box will be checked for insurance companies that require generic drugs to be dispensed unless the prescriber specifies dispense as written (DAW) on the prescription.

Check this box.

14   Check the **OTC Covered** box if over-the-counter (OTC) drugs are covered under this insurance plan.

OTC drugs are covered under this plan.

15   **Cost Prefs #1**, **#2**, and **#3** (cost preferences) are the three choices for calculating the ingredient cost of the drug. For each preference, the available choices are displayed in a pick list. Click the **Arrow** to the right of the data entry field to access the pick list. Select the three cost preferences. When pricing a prescription, Visual SuperScript first attempts to calculate the ingredient cost based on **Cost Prefs #1**. If **Cost Prefs #1** is unavailable (as indicated by a zero in that field in the drug record), Visual SuperScript then uses **Cost Prefs #2**, and so on.

Enter *AWP* (average wholesale price) as Cost Pref #1.
Enter *MAC* (manufacturers' average cost) as Cost Pref #2.
Enter *Direct* as Cost Pref #3.

16   Tab to the **Usual & Cust Charges?** data entry field. Click on the **Arrow** located to the right of the data entry field. Four options are provided on a drop-down list. Click on the desired name from the drop-down list.

Select *All Drugs* from the list.

Note: The **Usual & Cust Charges?** data entry field indicates whether the insurance company requires you to submit the usual and customary charges if the pharmacy's price of the medication is lower than the price based on the ingredient cost–plus–dispensing fee formula specified by the insurance company.

17   Click on the yellow tab entitled *Pricing Parameters*. The *Pricing Parameters* form is active and ready for data entry.

18   Key in the desired markup factor in the **BRAND MARKUP** data entry field.

> **Note:** The **BRAND MARKUP** is the factor by which the AWP (or MAC or direct cost) of the drug is multiplied to arrive at the ingredient cost of the drug for billing purposes. For example, a 10% markup should be entered as 1.1. A 100% markup should be entered as 2.00.

Enter *1* as the BRAND MARKUP.

19   Key in the **BRAND DISP FEE** allowed by the insurance company.

Enter *$3.50* as the BRAND DISP FEE.

> **Note:** The **BRAND DISP FEE** data entry field contains the dispensing fee allowed by the insurance company for brand-name drugs. The dispensing fee is added to the ingredient cost to arrive at the price of the drug.

20   Key in the markup factor for brand-name OTC drugs in the **BRAND MARKUP FOR OTC** data entry field.

Enter *1.25* as the BRAND MARKUP FOR OTC.

21   Key in the amount of money to be paid by the customer (copay) for each brand-name prescription in the **BRAND COPAY** data entry field.

Enter *20* as the BRAND COPAY.

> **Note:** The pharmacy collects the copay amount from the customer at the time the prescription is picked up from the pharmacy.

22   Check the **IS IT PERCENT?** box if the figure entered in the copay field is to be treated as a percentage of the price rather than an absolute dollar amount. For example, if the price of the drug is $45.00 and there is an entry of 10 in the copay field and the **IS IT PERCENT?** box is not checked, the copay computed by the system would be a $10.00 flat copay fee. However, if the **IS IT PERCENT?** box is checked, the copay will be computed as $4.50 (10% of $45.00).

Leave the *IS IT PERCENT?* box unchecked.

23   The **BRAND DISCOUNT COPAY** data entry field should reflect the same copay as the corresponding *Brand Copay* field *unless* your pharmacy has decided to offer a lower copay amount than required by the insurance company.

Key in the correct BRAND DISCOUNT COPAY as *20*, and leave IS IT PERCENT? information blank.

24   Key in the required information in the second column of the *Pricing Parameters* form. The second column is entitled **GENERIC**.

Generic Markup: 1

Generic Disp. Fee: $3.50

Generic Markup for OTC: $1.25

Generic Copay: $5

Generic Is It Percent? No

Generic Discount Copay: $5

Generic Is It Percent? No

25   Tab to the **SAME COPAY AS GENERICS FOR BRAND DRUGS WITH NO GEN** field. Check this box if the copay amounts for brand-name and generic drugs are different and the insurance company allows the customer to pay the same copay for generic drugs as it does for brand-name drugs that have no generic drugs available.

Check the SAME COPAY as Generics box.

Note: Usually, lower copay amounts are required for generic drugs versus brand-name drugs as an incentive for patients to choose generic over brand-name drugs. Under some plans, the customer is allowed to pay the lower copay amount when a drug has no generic drug available.

26   Tab to the **MAX PAYMENT FOR AN RX** field. This field specifies the maximum amount the insurance company will pay for a single prescription.

Enter a large value such as *9999* if no limit exists.

27   The **PERC. OF COST DIFF. BETWEEN BRAND & GENERICS PAIN** field specifies the *percentage* of the difference between the price of the brand-name drug and the price of the generic drug that the insurance company requires the patient to pay if the patient chooses a brand-name over the generic drug. Enter the correct percentage difference in the **PERC. OF COST DIFF. BETWEEN BRAND & GENERICS PAIN** field (see the screen shot on the following page).

Enter 80% ($80.00) as the percentage of cost difference.

HINT: See the screen shot on the next page for a sample of the **PRICING PARAMETERS** screen.

28 Click on the **ELECTRONIC BILLING OPTIONS** tab. The *Electronic Billing Options* form is active and ready for data entry.

Note: The information contained in the **ELECTRONIC BILLING OPTIONS** form determines to whom claims are sent for adjudication, as well as the format in which they are sent. Successful adjudication requires that all items must be entered as completely and accurately as possible.

29 The **EL. BILLER** (electronic biller) data entry field specifies the company to which the electronic claim is delivered initially. Click on the **COMBO-BOX DOWN ARROW** located to the right of the **EL. BILLER** data entry field. A dialog box entitled *Insurance Carrier* pops up. Select the appropriate company from the table by clicking on the company name. Then click **OK** located at the bottom of the *Insurance Carrier* dialog box.

Select *National Data Corp.* as the insurance carrier.

30 The **BIN** identifies the party to whom the electronic biller (from step 29) needs to forward the claim. This field is required for all electronically transmitted plans. Most insurance companies will list the **BIN** on the insurance card issued to the customer. The **BIN** always consists of six numeric characters. Key in the correct **BIN**.

Enter *510455* as the BIN.

31 The **Proc. Ctrl. #** (processing control number [PCS]) field is a required field for all electronically transmitted plans. The PCS may also be referred to as the *Carrier ID*. Key in the appropriate *Carrier ID*.

Enter *HCS* as the PCS/Carrier ID.

32 Tab to the **Required Prescriber MD ID** (required medical doctor or prescriber identification number) data entry field. Click on the **Arrow** located to the right of the data entry field. Select and click on the appropriate identification number type that the insurance company uses to identify the prescriber. For successful adjudication, selecting the appropriate identifier for each specific plan is imperative.

Select *DEA#* as the identifier.

33 Click on the **Combo-Box Down Arrow** located to the right of the **Default Other Coverage Code** data entry field. Click on the appropriate coverage code from the table in the *Default Other Coverage Code* dialog box. Click **OK** located at the bottom of the dialog box.

Select *0—Not Specified* as the code.

34 Click on the **Combo-Box Arrow** located to the right of the **Default Oth Code for Secondary Billing** data entry field. Click on the appropriate coverage code from the table in the *Default Other Coverage Code* dialog box. Click **OK** located at the bottom of the dialog box.

Select *0—Not Specified* as the code.

35 Click on the **Combo-Box Arrow** located to the right of the **Default Rx Origin Code** data entry field. Indicate if the third-party payer (e.g., insurance company) requires prescriptions to be written (select *1—Written Prescription*) or if the third-party payer has no preference on the form or origin of the prescription (select *0—Not Specified*). After choosing the correct prescription origin code, click **OK** located at the bottom of the *Rx Origin Code* dialog box.

Select *0—Not Specified* as the code.

36 Click on the **Combo-Box Arrow** located on the right side of the **Default Rx Denial Override Code** data entry field. Select the correct denial override code from the table in the dialog box. Click **OK** located on the bottom of the *Denial Override Code* dialog box.

Select *00—Not Specified* as the code.

37 Tab to the right side of the *Electronic Billing Options* form. Click on the **Combo-Box Arrow** located on the right side of the **Default Rx Elig Clar Code** data entry field. Select the correct prescription eligibility clarification code from the table in the dialog box. Click **OK** located on the bottom of the *Rx Elig Clar Code* dialog box.

Select *0—Not Specified* as the code.

38 The check boxes located on the right side of the *Electronic Billing Options* form are optional fields. Completion of these fields may be required for some insurance plans. To ensure proper adjudication of your claims, calling the insurance help desk to find out which fields are required may be necessary. Check the appropriate boxes.

> **Check the XMIT MULTIPLE CLAIMS (transmit multiple claims) check box to allow for transmitting multiple claims in a single transaction. If this check box is not checked, claims will be transmitted one at a time. In addition, check the Medicaid box.**

39 Click on the **SAVE** 🖫 icon located at the top of the *Insurance Plans* form. The insurance plan has now been added to the database.

40 Print the screen by using the **PRINTSCRN** option on your keyboard: Press the **PRINTSCRN** key, open a blank Word document, **RIGHT CLICK** the blank Word document, and then select **PASTE**.

Questions for Review

1 It is best to associate an insurance plan name with the name of the insurance company.

   a True

   b False

2 A pharmacy benefits manager is the entity who may process insurance claims for the insurance company.

   a True

   b False

3 The three tab names on the *Insurance Plans* form are

   _____, _____,

   and _____.

4 The IDENTIFICATION QUALIFIER is:

   a A coded number that identifies the insurance company

   b Used to identify the prescriber for third-party billing

   c The same for every plan

   d An optional data entry field

5 BILLING METHOD choices include:

   a Electronic billing

   b Universal claim form

   c Fax

   d Both a and b

6 The MAX REFILLS data entry field represents the:

   a Maximum number of refills the pharmacy will allow the patient to have

   b Maximum number of refills the insurance plan will allow the patient to have

   c Number of times the insurance company will pay on a given prescription to be refilled

   d Maximum number of refills the prescriber will allow the patient to have

7 Does your state impose a sales tax on prescription medications?

   a Yes

   b No

8   The copay amount for brand-name medications should always be marked as a percentage of the price of the medication.
   a True
   b False

9   An example of a third-party payer is the patient's insurance company.
   a True
   b False

10   The information contained in the *Electronic Billing Options* form determines:
   a To whom claims are sent for adjudication
   b The format in which claims are sent
   c Both a and b.
   d Patient copay amount only

11   The *Electronic Billing Options* form will be active only if the billing method choice is electronic billing.
   a True
   b False

12   The processing control number may also be referred to as the

   _____ or the _____.

13   The BIN:
   a Identifies the party to whom the electronic biller needs to forward the claim
   b Is a required field for all electronically transmitted plans
   c Is a six-digit number on the customer's insurance card
   d Is all of the above

14   NCPDP:
   a Is the official standard for pharmacy claims in the Health Insurance Portability and Accountability Act (HIPAA)
   b Is the National Council for Prescription Drug Programs
   c Provides pharmacies with a unique identifying number for interactions with federal agencies and third-party processors
   d Is all of the above

Exercise

Scenario

The pharmacy manager has asked you to update the database by adding a new insurance plan. Adding the new plan by the end of the day is important to submit a patient's prescription claim electronically. Your manager provides you with a detailing of the pricing information:

Pharmacy ID: 6503829
Brand markup is 1.5 (Rx and OTC)
The pharmacy offers a discount only for generic drug copay: 1%

Task

Use the following insurance plan information, as well as the information that the managing pharmacist has provided, to add an insurance plan to the database. Select *Not Specified* for any insurance information that is not provided. Submit each tabbed area of the *Insurance Plans* form on completion.

Insurance Plan Information

Plan Name: SureWay

Plan Details: The maximum number of refills allowed is 12. The maximum number of days supply is 32. Refills are allowed for a maximum of 1 year. The pharmacy should always dispense generic medications unless otherwise indicated by the physician. If a generic medication is not available, the customer will pay the generic copay amount for brand-name medications. If a generic medication is available but the customer prefers the brand-name medication, the customer must pay 90% of the price cost difference between the brand and generic drugs. All medications are subject to usual and customary charges. OTC drugs are not covered under this plan.

Company Name: SystemED
ID Qualifier: NCPDP—Format version 3A
Electronic Biller: Pro-Serv
BIN: 610053
Processor Control: 7Q 7700970
Cost Preference: AWP
Dispensing Fees: $3.00 brand/generic
Flat Copay Amounts: $10.00 Brand/$2.50 generic
Maximum Payment: None
Prescriber Qualifier: DEA number
Note: A code is required for claim reversal.

Adding a Drug to the Database and Other Inventory Tasks

LAB OBJECTIVES

In this lab, you will:

- Add a new drug to the database by National Drug Code (NDC) number.
- Visually identify a drug by using the database.
- Adjust the ordering quantities of a drug.

STUDENT DIRECTIONS

Estimated completion time: 30 minutes

1. Read through the steps in the lab before performing the lab exercise.
2. After reading through the lab, perform the required steps to enter the new drug to the database.
3. Complete the exercise at the end of the lab.

Steps to Add a Drug to the Database

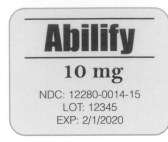

Use the above drug label to complete the following steps.

1 Access the main screen of Visual SuperScript.

2 Click on the **DRUG** button located on the left side of the screen. A dialog box appears entitled *Drugs*. This *Drugs* form is used to maintain a database of drugs that are dispensed in the pharmacy.

3 Click on **ADD DRUGS BY NDC** located at the top left side of the form. A dialog box entitled *Add Drug by NDC* appears.

NDC	Drug Name	Strength	Package Size	Manufacturer	Obselete Date	
00002-0604-40	SEROMYCIN 250 MG PULVULE	250 MG	40.000	ELI LILLY & CO.	06/01/2009	
00002-1407-01	QUINIDINE GLUC 80 MG/ML VIAL	80 MG/ML	10.000	ELI LILLY & CO.	/ /	
00002-1485-01	CAPASTAT SULFATE 1 GM VIAL	1 G	1.000	ELI LILLY & CO.	07/17/2009	
00002-3004-75	PROZAC WEEKLY 90 MG CAPSULE	90 MG	4.000	ELI LILLY & CO.	/ /	
00002-3145-30	AXID 300 MG PULVULE	300 MG	30.000	ELI LILLY & CO.	08/18/2008	
00002-3227-30	STRATTERA 10 MG CAPSULE	10 MG	30.000	ELI LILLY & CO.	/ /	
00002-3228-30	STRATTERA 25 MG CAPSULE	25 MG	30.000	ELI LILLY & CO.	/ /	
00002-3229-30	STRATTERA 40 MG CAPSULE	40 MG	30.000	ELI LILLY & CO.	/ /	
00002-3230-30	SYMBYAX 3-25 MG CAPSULE	3MG-25MG	30.000	ELI LILLY & CO.	/ /	
00002-3231-01	SYMBYAX 6-25 MG CAPSULE	6MG-25MG	100.000	ELI LILLY & CO.	/ /	

Add Drug By NDC — NDC [- -] — Obselete Date 06/21/2008

[Add Drug] [Cancel]

4 Key in the NDC number as it appears on the stock bottle label.

Type *12280-0014-15* for Abilify 10 mg.

5 Select the appropriate entry by clicking on the correct NDC number.

6 Click on **ADD DRUG** located at the bottom of the dialog box.

7 The *Drugs* form has now been updated with the new medication. Click on the **EDIT** 📝 icon located on the bottom right of the form.

8 The *Drug NDC* dialog box appears. Tab to the **LOT #** data entry field on the right side of the dialog box. Key in the drug lot number according to the stock bottle label.

Type *12345* for the lot number.

9   Click on the **SAVE** button at the bottom of the *Drug NDC* dialog box.

10   Click on the **EDIT** 📝 icon located at the top of the *Drugs* form.

11   Tab to the **QUICK CODES** data entry field. Enter the first few characters of the drug name in the **QUICK CODES** data entry field.

Enter *ABL10* into this field.

> **HINT: QUICK CODES** allow you to expedite the search for drugs when filling perscriptions.

Note: The **ALCHEMY PRODUCT ID** field is automatically completed with the selection of the drug if an ID is assigned to the drug. In the practice setting, completing the entry in this field is important because this code produces all warning and counseling messages for the drug. Many other data entry fields are also automatically completed with the selection of the drug. The **DRUG CLASS**, **ITEM TYPE**, **GENDER**, and **BRAND/GENERIC** fields have been updated to coincide with the drug selection.

12   Tab to the **DEFAULT SIG** data entry field.

Enter the sig abbreviation *T 1 T PO QD* for "Take one tablet by mouth once daily" for Abilify instructions.

Note: Certain drugs are frequently prescribed with the same instructions for use. Entering the appropriate instructions in the **DEFAULT SIG** field can save time when filling a prescription.

13   Tab to the **MAX DOSE** data entry field. Key in the maximum daily dose advised for this particular medication.

Enter *2* as the maximum dose for Abilify.

14   Tab to the **DEFAULT QUANTITY** data entry field. Certain drugs are frequently prescribed with the same quantity instructions. Key in the desired quantity to be dispensed in the prescription for this particular medication.

Enter *30* as the default quantity for Abilify.

15   Tab to the **DEFAULT DAY SUPPLY** data entry field, and key in the desired quantity.

Enter *30*.

16 Click the yellow **PRICING AND STOCK** tab located at the top of the form.

Note: The **PRICE TABLE** is a required field that links each drug to a pricing formula for the purpose of calculating the usual and customary price of the drug. The correct **PRICE TABLE** has automatically been added with the selection of the drug.

17 Click on the **EXPIRE DATE** (expiration date) data entry field. Key in the drug expiration date according to the stock bottle label.

Enter 02/01/2020

18 Tab to the area of the form entitled *Track Inventory*. Key in the **MINIMUM STOCK** value that the pharmacy wishes to maintain for the new medication that is being added to the database.

Enter 90 for MINIMUM STOCK.

19 In the **REORDER QTY.** (reorder quantity) data entry field, key in the quantity of medication that the pharmacy will reorder when the stock is at its minimum.

Enter *60* for reorder quantity.

20 Key in the actual amount or quantity of medication that will be added to the pharmacy shelf in the **LAST VERIFIED STOCK** data entry field.

Four stock bottles of Abilify will be added to the pharmacy shelf. Each bottle contains 30 tablets. Therefore key in *120* in the verified stock data entry field.

Note: The **LAST VERIFIED STOCK** field is the amount of drug that is being added to the pharmacy shelf. This amount could be tablets, capsules, or liquid form (milliliters).

> **LAB TIP:** VERIFICATION DATE is the date that the new drug is being added to the pharmacy shelf, and is automatically populated.

Note: The pink tab, **WELFARE & MISC**, located at the top of the form is not used for all drugs. This tab will be used when working with controlled substances and special considerations for Medicaid.

21 Click on the **SAVE** 🖫 icon located at the top of the *Drugs* form. The new drug has now been added to the pharmacy's working drug file.

22 Click on the **CLOSE** 🗗 icon located at the top of the *Drugs* form.

Exercise

Using the invoice for an order received in the pharmacy and your data entry skills, add Advil 200 mg to the pharmacy inventory. Appropriately apply stickers on the bottles. On completion of this exercise, submit the screenshots, stock bottles, and invoice for verification.

Quick Challenge

1 You have learned how to add drugs to the software database. In reading the steps in this lab, you have come to understand that the pharmacy will order and update stock on a regular basis. Can you complete an electronic purchase order for ordering medication stock for the pharmacy?

2 Order the following stock from XYZ Drugs, Inc. Print the purchase order and submit for verification.
- Reorder Quantity: 56-Prempro 0.625/2.5 mg tab #00046-0875-6
- Reorder Quantity: 200-Synthroid 125 mcg #00048-1130-03
- Reorder Quantity: 90-Nexium 20 mg capsule #00186-5020-31

Steps to Adjust the Reorder Quantities for a Drug

1 Access the main screen of Visual SuperScript.

2 Click on the **DRUG** button located on the left side of the screen. A dialog box appears entitled *Drugs*.

3 Click on the **FIND** 🔍 icon at the top left of the *Drugs* dialog box.

4 Type in the first three letters of the drug to search and click **OK** to select the correct drug and dosage.

Type *Zit* for Zithromax 250 mg z-pak tablet.

5 Click on the yellow **PRICING AND STOCK** tab located at the top of the form.

6 Click on the **EDIT** 📝 icon at the top of the screen, and edit the following stock data fields:

Change the MINIMUM STOCK to *24*
and the REORDER QUANTITY to *48*.

7 Click on the **SAVE** 💾 icon located at the top of the *Drugs* form. The new drug has now been added to the pharmacy's working drug file.

8 Click on the **CLOSE** 🔌 icon located at the top of the *Drugs* form.

Steps to Verify Drug Identity

You have learned how to add new drugs to the software database, as well as change the order amount. In practice, a visual identification of a drug is required at times.

1 Access the main screen of Visual SuperScript.

2 Click on the **DRUG** button located on the left side of the screen. A dialog box appears entitled *Drugs*.

3 Click on the **FIND** 🔍 icon at the top left of the *Drugs* dialog box.

4   Type in the first three letters of the drug to search and click **OK** to select the correct drug and dosage.

Type *Lex* for Lexapro 20 mg tablets.

5   On the bottom right hand side of the screen, click on the **EDIT** button, and a box called *Drug NDC* will appear that gives a general description of the medication.

LAB TIP: The **EDIT** button used for drug image is at the bottom of the screen, not the one at the top of the *Drugs* box.

6   Choose the **DRUG IMAGE** button on the bottom left of the *Drug NDC* box for an image of the medication.

Exercise

Mrs. Brown is an older patient who lives alone and often brings her "brown bag" of medication to the pharmacy for identification. Use the **DRUG IMAGE** lab and the profile list below of her medications to give her a description of each medication.

- Prevacid 30 mg capsule
- Tegretol 200 mg tablets
- Risperdal 2 mg tablets
- Neurontin 300 mg capsule

Print a screen shot of the image window for each drug for this assignment.

Entering a New Prescription

LAB OBJECTIVES

In this lab, you will:

- Learn how to perform necessary computer functions to enter a new prescription into a pharmacy system.
- Learn about dispense as written (DAW) codes.
- Learn shortcuts to be used when entering sigs.

STUDENT DIRECTIONS

Estimated completion time: 10 minutes

1. Read through the steps in the lab before performing the lab exercise.
2. After reading through the lab, perform the required steps to create a label and prepare the product for dispensing.
3. Complete the exercise at the end of the lab.

Pre Lab Information

Regardless of the practice setting for the pharmacy technician and pharmacist, entering data into the computer is a major component of their workload. In the retail setting, for example, a customer drops off the prescription hard copy. After the pharmacy technician has obtained all the necessary information from the customer, information is entered into the computer. This lab explains the steps involved in filling new prescriptions.

Working through the steps involved in interpreting and transcribing a prescription is beneficial before completing the following lab.

Steps to Enter a New Prescription

> # R_x
>
> **Dr. John Thompson**
> **81 Highland Street**
> **Allston, MA 02134**
> **Office: (617) 632-4568**
> **Fax: (617) 734-6340**
>
> ---
>
> **Patient Name:** Karen Anderson
>
> **Date:** 2/17/2012
>
> **Address:**   526 Maple Street, Wellesby, MA
>
> Refill: 2
> Rx: Lipitor 40 mg, 1 hs #30
> Brand Necessary
>
> ---
>
> **DEA:** AT4278431
> **State License:** 3445542

Use the above prescription to complete the following steps.

1 Access the main menu of Visual SuperScript.

2 Click on **FILL RX'S** located on the left side of the menu screen. The *Prescription Processing* form appears.

3 Click on the **NEW RX** icon on the top left of the *Prescription Processing* form.

   Note: Prescription information such as the **RX NO.** (prescription number) and **DISPENSE DATE** are automatically generated and added to the form. You may also choose the **RX ORIGIN** from the drop-down menu if the prescription is not written.

4 Enter your initials in the *Enter Tech Init* box that appears and click **OK**.

5 You will then be prompted to the **CUSTOMER'S LOOKUP** (highlighted in blue) text box. Type the first three letters of the last name and hit **ENTER**.

   Type *AND* for Karen Anderson
   as indicated in the sample prescription.

6 Select the appropriate customer by double-clicking on the customer name or by clicking **OK**.

Note: The customer's personal information such as **ADDRESS**, **PHONE**, and **BIRTHDATE** will be automatically added to the *Prescription Processing* form.

Note: You are automatically directed to the **DOCTOR** text box once the patient information is populated. For new prescriptions, the system will search the patient's prescription file to find the name of the prescriber of the most recently filled prescription. If found, the system will insert the prescriber's name into this field. If a different doctor has written the new prescription, you can delete the old name and enter a new one. For this particular exercise, the physician, Dr. John Thompson, is listed in the sample prescription and is automatically populated in this field.

7   Press the **TAB** key. You will be prompted to the **PRESCRIBED DRUG** data entry field. Key in the first three letters of the prescribed drug into the **PRESCRIBED DRUG** data entry field. Then press **ENTER**.

ENTER *Lip* for Karen Anderson's Lipitor.

8   Select the appropriate drug entitled *Drug Name Lookup* from the drop-down list by double-clicking on the drug name.

> **LAB TIP:** If a series of warning dialog boxes appear, these are known as drug utilization reviews (DURs). The patient's medication history is compared against the drug you are entering for pregnancy warnings, drug-drug and drug-food interactions, or contraindication conditions or diseases. (The warning messages should be viewed and approved by the pharmacist before dispensing the medication.)

9   After receiving approval from the Instructor to continue, click the **CLOSE** 🚪 icon to move through the warnings. Click **CONTINUE RX** to navigate to the next step.

10   Drug information such as **NDC#** and **MANUFACTURER** will appear under **AVAILABLE DRUG CHOICE**. Choose the generic substitution unless the doctor has specified, "dispense as written" (DAW).

11   Next, you will be prompted to the **REFILLS ORDERED** data entry field. Key in the appropriate number of refills.

12   Press the **TAB** key. You will be prompted to enter the prescribed quantity. Key in the appropriate quantity in the **PRESCRIBED QUANTITY** data entry field.

13 Press the **TAB** key until you reach the **DAW** text box. Choose the correct **DAW** code by clicking on the **ARROW** on the right side of the **DAW** data entry field.

Click on the correct DAW code from the pick list.

Note: When filling a prescription, knowing the correct **DAW** code to be assigned to a prescription is necessary for reimbursement. For this to be accomplished, distinguish between the brand name and the generic name of the medication. Although the prescriber may write the brand name of a drug on a patient's prescription, it may not necessarily mean that the brand-name drug must be dispensed. If the prescriber indicates **DAW** or "brand name medically necessary" on the patient's prescription for a brand-name drug, then the brand-name drug rather than the generic alternative MUST be dispensed. This situation, for example, would be a **DAW** code 1. The failure to use the proper **DAW** codes may result in improper third-party reimbursement to the pharmacy. Seven **DAW** codes are used in the pharmacy practice:

DAW 0—Physician has approved the dispensing of a generic medication.

DAW 1—Physician requests that the brand-name drug be dispensed.

DAW 2—Physician has approved the dispensing of a generic drug, but the patient has requested that the brand-name drug be dispensed.

DAW 3—Pharmacist dispenses the drug as written.

DAW 4—No generics are available in the store.

DAW 5—Brand-name drug is dispensed but priced as a generic drug.

DAW 6—RPh doctor call is attempted.

14 Press the **TAB** key. Key in the patient abbreviated directions in the **SIG** text box.

**Key in *T1T PO HS* as the shortcut abbreviation sig
for Karen Anderson.**

Note: What appears in the blue **SIG IN ENGLISH** space is what will appear on the label. If an error is made when typing in the sig, backspace to delete the error and retype the correct information.

15   Press the **TAB** key. You will be prompted to enter **PRESCRIBED DAYS SUPPLY**. Key in the appropriate days supply in the **PRESCRIBED DAYS SUPPLY** data entry field.

ENTER *30* for Karen Anderson's days supply.

Note: Days supply involves calculating the number of days that a particular prescription will last. All third-party payers require this information. The failure to provide days supply information properly may result in the pharmacy losing money. To calculate the days supply a prescription will last, use the following formula:

$$\text{Days supply} = \frac{\text{Total quantity dispensed}}{\text{Total quantity taken per day}}$$

The days supply is the number of days a medication will last for one filling. Days supply does not take into account refills. The majority of the third-party payers will reimburse a pharmacy for a 30-day supply of medication.

Note: You may tab back to the **RX NOTES** section and add any notes that apply. Most states require patients to receive the opportunity for medication counseling. The **RX NOTES** section is a good spot to document "offered counseling, but patient refused counseling" or other similar important information.

16   Press the **ENTER** key. You are now prompted to save the prescription information. Click the **SAVE** 🖫 icon .

HINT: Make sure you save using the **SAVE** button to the right. (Save this Rx in the System Memory.) Visual SuperScript will default to the **SAVE** button on the left, which will save the entry and automatically move you to a new prescription for the same customer. If you use the **SAVE** button on the left and the screen goes blank, then you can click the **BACK** button to reclaim the Rx and print the label.

17 Click on **LABEL** on the left of the screen to complete adjudication and **PRINT**.

18 Prepare the medication for dispensing, including labeling the product. Affix the second label to the back of the original prescription.

Exercise

Enter prescriptions and prepare products for dispensing using the assigned prescriptions found in Appendix B. Leave the stock bottle, original prescription, and prepared product for a pharmacist final check. Remember to affix the second label on the back of the original prescription in your book.

Note: Practice using the abbreviation shortcuts found in Appendix A to make the process quicker. All drug community software programs use these abbreviations to save time. Some prescriptions may require adding new patient information, new prescriber information, or adding a new drug to the database. You may review Section 1 for these procedures.

Maxine Braswell
Pg 150

Obtaining a Refill Authorization

LAB OBJECTIVES

In this lab, you will:

- Learn how to refill a prescription by number or customer name.
- Create a new prescription out of an expired prescription.
- Learn the procedure for faxing the prescriber for additional refill requests.

STUDENT DIRECTIONS

Estimated completion time: 20 minutes

1. Read through the steps in the lab before performing the lab exercise.
2. After reading through the lab, perform the required steps for a refill or prepare a *Refill Authorization* request.
3. Answer the questions at the end of the lab.
4. Complete the exercise at the end of the lab.

Steps for Refilling a Prescription Using a Prescription Number

1 Access the main screen of Visual SuperScript.

2 Click on **OPTIONS** on the top right of the menu screen, and select **WORKSTATION SETUP**. Make sure your printer is selected in the **LABEL PRINTER** field.

Workstation Setup

☑ Use Internet to Send Claims   Signature Capture Port [0]

Comm Port [3] Baud Rate [38400] [⬇] Dial Prefix [9,]

Fax Class [CLASS 2.0 ▼]   Dial Suffix [ ]

[Detect Fax Modem]

[Label Printer] [\\server\Lexmark C910 PS3]

Paper Source [Auto Select]   Size [Letter 8 1/2 x 11 in]

Left Margin [0.00 ⬍]   Top Margin [0.00 ⬍]

[Report Printer] [SHARP AR-M237 PCL6 (Tray 2)]

Paper Source [Auto Select]   ☐ Prompt Printer

Left Margin [0.00 ⬍]   Top Margin [0.00 ⬍]

[Fax Printer] [Vissuper FaxPrinter]

[Install Fax Printer]

[Scanner] [ ]

Rx Size [Quarter-Page]

[OK] [Cancel]

---

3 Click the **FILL RX'S** button on the left side of the main menu.

4   The *Prescription Processing* form appears on your screen. Click on the **REFILL BY RX#** button located on the left side of the screen. Clicking on the **ARROW** next to the **REFILL RX'S** menu on the left of the form may be necessary to access the choices on the expanded **REFILL RX'S** menu.

5   Key in the prescription number that is to be refilled in the **Rx No.** box.

Enter *201268* as the prescription refill number.

6   The *Cannot Refill, Select Copy Options* dialog box appears. This dialog box will appear when a prescription has no refills remaining or if the prescription has expired.

Note: Refill authorizations are usually requested for maintenance or for routine prescriptions for a customer. A technician may process a refill once the authorization form is returned from the physician as long as no changes have occurred, and this document becomes a new prescription with the new date.

7   Click on ~~**PRINT**~~ Preview **REFILL AUTH REQUEST FORM** located on the right side of the dialog box to generate, and print the *Refill Authorization Form* for the patient's medication. This *Refill Authorization Form* may then be printed or faxed to the patient's physician.

Steps for Refilling a Prescription Once the Refill Authorization Has Been Granted

1   Access the main screen of Visual SuperScript.

2   Click on **OPTIONS** on the top right of the menu screen, and select **WORKSTATION SETUP**. Make sure your printer is selected.

3   Click the **FILL RX'S** button on the left side of the main menu.

4   The *Prescription Processing* form appears on your screen. Click on the **REFILL BY RX#** button located on the left side of the screen. Clicking on the **ARROW** next to the **REFILL RX'S** menu on the left of the form may be necessary to access the choices on the expanded **REFILL RX'S** menu choices.

5   Key in the prescription number that is to be refilled in the **Rx No.** box.

Enter *201268* as the prescription refill number.

6   Click on **COPY TO NEW RX** pad located on the right of the *Cannot Refill, Select Copy Options* dialog box.

7   A series of dialog boxes will appear alerting you to *Price Increases* and/or *HIPAA*-related information. Navigate through these dialog boxes by clicking on **OK**, **CLOSE**, or **YES**. The *Prescription Processing* form appears, and a new prescription is automatically created. The number of authorized subsequent refills will need to be added to the prescription according to the returned **AUTH REQUEST FORM**.

8   Make note that the new prescription number and other prescription information is automatically added to the form.

9   Click on the **SAVE** 🖫 icon located at the top left of the screen.

10   Click on **LABEL** at the top left of the form.

Steps to Refilling a Prescription Using a Patient's Name

1   Access the main screen of Visual SuperScript.

2   Click on **OPTIONS** on the top right of the menu screen, and select **WORKSTATION SETUP**. Make sure your printer is selected.

3   Select **FILL RX'S** on the menu screen on the left. Then click on the **CUS HISTORY/REFILL** button on the left side of the dialog box.

4   The *Customer History: Refill Rx* dialog screen will appear. Click on the *Prescriptions on File* (yellow) tab. Type in the first three letters of the customer's name to perform a search.

Enter *DAV* for Nancy Davis.

Mrs. Davis has called in a refill for her Albuterol inhaler Rx# 386553.

Customer History: Refill Rx's

| Customer | | | | Phone ( ) - | | Refill Rx | Cancel | | User Interface ◉ Basic ○ Advance |
| Address | | | | Birthdate | | | | | |

Prescriptions on File | Refill History

R	Rx #	Pres Date ↑	Prescribed Drug	Quantity	Days Supply	Rem. Qty	Rem. Days	Last Fill Date	Last Disp. Qty	Doctor

Hot Keys | M= Menu | A= Show All | D= Show Selected Drug Only | R= Selected for Refills | H= Refill History | F= Fill Rx
S= Sort On Prescribed / Dispensed Date | E= Edit Prescription | I= Inactivate Rx | T= Transfer Rx Out

Show All | Selected Drug | Selected For Refills | Drug

5   Enter a check in the blank on the left side of the screen by using the mouse. Click on **REFILL RX'S** at the top right of the dialog screen.

Customer History: Refill Rx's

| Customer | DAVIS, NANCY | | | Phone (617) 638-4271 | | Refill Rx | Cancel | | User Interface ◉ Basic ○ Advance |
| Address | 14 RUSSELL STREET | | | Birthdate 12/14/1951 | | | | | |

Prescriptions on File= 5 , # Selected for Refills= 1 | Refill History

R	Rx #	Pres Date ↑	Prescribed Drug	Quantity	Days Supply	Rem. Qty	Rem. Days	Last Fill Date	Last Disp. Qty	Doctor
	387465	05/27/2009	METOPROLOL 25 MG TABLET	60.000	30	300.000		05/27/2009	60.000	MARTINEZ, PAUL A.
	386869	04/16/2005	NAPROXEN 500 MG TABLET EC	90.000	30	180.000		04/16/2005	90.000	MARTINEZ, PAUL A.
	386613	02/02/2005	PREDNISONE 5 MG TABLET	30.000	30	90.000		04/03/2005	30.000	MARTINEZ, PAUL A.
✓	386553	01/16/2005	ALBUTEROL 90 MCG INHALER	17.000	30	136.000		04/16/2005	17.000	HARDY, STEPHEN
	386552	01/16/2005	ALLEGRA 60 MG CAPSULE	30.000	30	240.000		04/16/2005	30.000	HARDY, STEPHEN

Hot Keys | M= Menu | A= Show All | D= Show Selected Drug Only | R= Selected for Refills | H= Refill History | F= Fill Rx
S= Sort On Prescribed / Dispensed Date | E= Edit Prescription | I= Inactivate Rx | T= Transfer Rx Out

Show All | Selected Drug | Selected For Refills | Drug

6   Complete the processing of the refill by either completing an *Authorization Request Form* if required or refilling as a regular prescription.

Questions for Review

1 What is the sig on Joseph Price's prescription?

2 What company manufacturers the medication refilled in Joseph Price's prescription?

3 What are the price and copay on the Vasotec prescription for Joseph Price?

4 What is the new prescription number that was created for Joseph Price's prescription?

Exercise

1 Follow the steps from the preceding lab to refill the following medication orders. Submit the labels for verification.
- Brian Davidson's Pen-Vee K #201096
- Fred Flintstone's Demadex #386530

Processing a New Prescription for a Prior Drug Approval

LAB OBJECTIVES

In this lab, you will:

- Learn how to perform computer functions necessary to enter a new prescription into a pharmacy system for an approved prior drug.
- Understand what prior drug approval or nonformulary drugs require for processing.
- Perform the necessary documentation required for prior drug approval.

STUDENT DIRECTIONS

Estimated completion time: 20 minutes

1. Read through the steps in the lab before performing the lab exercise.
2. After reading through the lab, perform the required steps to create a label and prepare the product for dispensing.
3. Complete the exercise at the end of the lab.

Pre Lab Information

Physicians sometimes order medications that require additional justification because of cost, dosage, or medical necessity before a third-party insurance company will pay for them. When coverage is required for a drug that is not on the insurance company's list (nonformulary) or medical justification is required (prior approval), the pharmacy personnel and physician must complete documentation before the prescription can be processed. This process can be done online, as well as manually, and is part of the adjudication process. This lab explains the steps involved in filling a new prescription for a current prior drug approval.

> **LAB TIP:** Understanding the steps of adding a new prescription (see Lab 6) is essential before completing the following lab.

Steps to Process a New Prescription for a Prior-Approved Drug

---

Rx

Dr. J. Kennedy
1623 Camelot Drive
Brighton, MA 02135
Office: (617) 439-8800
Fax: (617) 734-6340

Patient Name: Larry Jones

Date: 2/17/2012

Address: 100 King Street, Boston, MA

Refill: 0
Rx: Celebrex 100 mg, 1 bid #60
Brand Necessary

DEA: AK6321892
State License: 2556321

Use the above prescription to complete the following steps.

1   Access the main menu of Visual SuperScript.

2   Click on **FILL RX'S** located on the left side of the menu screen. The *Prescription Processing* form appears.

3   Click on the **NEW RX** icon on the top left of the *Prescription Processing* form.

Note: Prescription information such as the **RX No.** (prescription number) and **DISPENSE DATE** are automatically generated and added to the form. You may also choose the **RX ORIGIN** from the drop-down menu if it is not written.

> **LAB TIP:** Enter your initials in the *Enter Tech Init* box if it appears and click **OK**.

4   You will then be prompted to the **CUSTOMER'S LOOKUP** (highlighted in blue) text box. Type the first three letters of the last name and hit **ENTER**.

Type *Jon* Larry Jones DOB (01/01/1901) as indicated in the sample Rx.

5   Select the appropriate customer by double-clicking on the customer name or by clicking **OK**.

Note: The customer's personal information such as **ADDRESS**, **PHONE**, and **BIRTHDATE** will be automatically added to the *Prescription Processing* form.

Note: You are automatically directed to the **DOCTOR** text box once the patient information is populated. For new prescriptions, the system will search the patient's prescription file to find the name of the prescriber of the most recently filled prescription. If found, the system will insert that name into this field. If a different doctor writes the new prescription, you can delete the old name and enter a new one. For this particular exercise, the physician, Dr. J. Kennedy, is listed in the sample prescription and is not automatically populated in this field.

Refer to your sample prescription and use Dr. J. Kennedy.

6   Press the **TAB** key. You will be prompted to the **PRESCRIBED DRUG** data entry field. Key in the first three letters of the prescribed drug into the **PRESCRIBED DRUG** data entry field. Then press **ENTER**.

ENTER *Cel* FOR CELEBREX 100 MG.

7   Select the appropriate drug entitled *Drug Name Lookup* from the drop-down list by double-clicking on the drug name.

> **LAB TIP:** If a series of warning dialog boxes appear, these are known as drug utilization reviews (DURs). The patient's medication history is compared against the drug you are entering for pregnancy warnings, drug-drug and drug-food interactions, or contraindication conditions or diseases. (The warning messages should be viewed and approved by the pharmacist before dispensing the medication.)

8   After receiving approval from the Instructor to continue, click the **CLOSE** icon to move through the warnings. Click **CONTINUE RX** to navigate to the next step.

9   Drug information such as **NDC#** and **MANUFACTURER** will appear under **AVAILABLE DRUG CHOICE**. Choose the generic substitution unless the doctor has specified "dispense as written" (DAW).

10   Next, you will be prompted to the **REFILLS ORDERED** data entry field. Key in the appropriate number of refills.

11   Press the **TAB** key. You will be prompted to enter the prescribed quantity. Key in the appropriate quantity in the **PRESCRIBED QUANTITY** data entry field.

12   Press the **TAB** key until you reach the **DAW** text box. Choose the correct **DAW** code by clicking on the **ARROW** on the right side of the **DAW** data entry field.

Click on the correct DAW code from the pick list.

Note: When filling a prescription, knowing the correct **DAW** code to be assigned to a prescription is necessary for reimbursement. For this to be accomplished, distinguish between the brand name and the generic name of the medication. Although the prescriber may write the brand name of a drug on a patient's prescription, it may not necessarily mean that the brand-name drug must be dispensed. If the prescriber indicates **DAW** or "brand name medically necessary" on the patient's prescription for a brand-name drug, then the brand-name drug rather than the generic alternative MUST be dispensed. This situation, for example, would be a **DAW** code 1. The failure to use the proper **DAW** codes may result in improper third-party reimbursement to the pharmacy. Seven **DAW** codes are used in the pharmacy practice:

DAW 0—Physician has approved the dispensing of a generic medication.

DAW 1—Physician requests that the brand-name drug be dispensed.

DAW 2—Physician has approved the dispensing of a generic drug, but the patient has requested that the brand-name drug be dispensed.

DAW 3—Pharmacist dispenses the drug as written.

DAW 4—No generics are available in the store.

DAW 5—Brand-name drug is dispensed but priced as a generic drug.

DAW 6—RPh doctor call is attempted.

13 Press the **TAB** key. Key in the patient abbreviated directions in the **SIG** text box.

> **Key in *1CBID* as the shortcut abbreviation sig for "Take one capsule twice each day."**

Note: What appears in the blue **SIG IN ENGLISH** space is what will appear on the label. If an error is made when typing in the sig, backspace to delete the error and retype the correct information.

14 Press the **TAB** key. You will be prompted to enter **PRESCRIBED DAYS SUPPLY**. Key in the appropriate days supply in the **PRESCRIBED DAYS SUPPLY** data entry field.

> **ENTER *30* for the days supply.**

Note: Days supply involves calculating the number of days that a particular prescription will last. All third-party payers require this information. The failure to provide days supply information properly may result in the pharmacy losing money. To calculate the days supply a prescription will last, use the following formula:

$$\text{Days supply} = \frac{\text{Total quantity dispensed}}{\text{Total quantity taken per day}}$$

The days supply is the number of days a medication will last for one filling. Days supply does not take into account refills. The majority of the third-party payers will reimburse a pharmacy for a 30-day supply of medication.

Note: You may tab back to the **Rx Notes** section and add any notes that apply. Most states require patients to receive the opportunity for medication counseling. The **Rx Notes** section is a good place to document "offered counseling, but patient refused" or other important information. Enter the following note: "Prior-approved drug request sent to physician, dated, and with your initials."

15 Press the **ENTER** key. Click the **SAVE** 🖫 icon .

16 Click on **LABEL** on the left of the screen to complete adjudication and **PRINT**.

17 Manually complete the Pharmacy section only of the *Prior Authorization* (PA) form for this drug.

18 A copy of the PA form, the prescription, and the pharmacy label will be filed until it returns with approval, usually in 24 to 48 hours. Once the approval is granted, the prescription will be filled for the patient.

19 For this exercise, print the prescription label and prepare the PA form for your instructor to check.

Exercise

Enter prescriptions and prepare a PA form for each drug, using the prescriptions and the blank PA form given to you by your instructor. Leave all documentation, original prescription, and prepared label for a pharmacist's final check.

Note: Practice using the abbreviation shortcuts found in Appendix A to make the process quicker. All drug community software programs use these abbreviations to save time. Some prescriptions may require adding new patient information, new prescriber information, or adding a new drug to the database. You may review Section 1 for these procedures.

Refilling, Transferring, Filing, and Prescription Reversal

LAB OBJECTIVES

In this lab, you will:

- Process a customer's set of refilled prescriptions.
- Perform the computer functions to transfer a prescription to another pharmacy.
- Complete the steps to put a prescription on file.
- Process a prescription reversal. (The Quick Challenge will guide you through this.)

STUDENT DIRECTIONS

Estimated completion time: 60 minutes

1. Read through the steps in the lab before performing the lab exercise.
2. After reading through the lab, perform the required steps to complete the tasks in each scenario.

Refilling Prescriptions by Customer Name

Scenario

Mr. Ronald Jackson asks you to refill all of his medications for January and February, 2005. He may not remember all of the names or all of his prescription numbers. You can use the customer profile to locate each one for refilling.

Task

Fill Ronald Jackson's 2005 medications.

Steps to Refill Ronald Jackson's 2005 Medications

Use the information in the above scenario to complete the following steps.

1 Access the main menu of Visual SuperScript.

2 Click on **FILL RX'S** located on the left side of the menu screen. The *Prescription Processing* form appears.

3 Click on **CUS HISTORY/REFILL**.

> **LAB TIP:** If necessary, click on the **ARROW** next to the **REFILL RX'S** menu on the left of the form to access the expanded **REFILL RX'S** menu.

4 Key the customer name into the **CUSTOMER** data entry field of the *Customer History: Refill Rx's* dialog box. Press the **ENTER** key. The *Customer Lookup* dialog box appears. Click on the correct customer from the list in the *Customer Lookup* dialog box. Click **OK**.

Enter customer name *JACKSON, RONALD*.

5 Select the tab titled **PRESCRIPTIONS OF FILE**. Put a checkmark in the check box of the prescriptions that need to be refilled.

6 Click on **REFILL RX** located at the top of the dialog box.

Note: If the prescription has *not* expired and refills are remaining, the *Prescription Processing* form is updated with the refill information and a label can be printed.

Note: If the prescription has expired or has no refills, follow the procedure in Lab 7 for obtaining a *Refill Authorization* request.

7 The *Prescription Processing* form now returns to the screen. All medications checked will be processed. Click on **LABEL** located at the top left of the form. Clicking on **LABEL** will prompt the software to adjudication.

Note: This educational version of Visual SuperScript will not allow adjudication. You will receive a message that electronic billing is not supported. Click **OK**. To print the labels, change the **PAY TYPE** to *Cash*.

Transferring a Prescription

Pre Lab Information

Patients often want their prescriptions transferred to another pharmacy because of convenience, costs, or travel situations. Each state has certain regulations, which may determine whether certain medications can be transferred in and out of a state, and these must be followed. If allowed, specific information must be shared between the corresponding pharmacies.

Scenario

Mrs. Shirley Jones telephones the pharmacy explaining that she is on vacation visiting her daughter in Phoenix, Arizona. Mrs. Jones is out of her Hyzaar. She requests that you give her Hyzaar prescription information to a nearby pharmacy in Phoenix that would enable her to refill her medication.

Task

Follow the "Steps to Transferring a Prescription" listed below to transfer Shirley Jones' prescription for Hyzaar to the following pharmacy:

Sun Drug
102 Indian School Rd.
Phoenix, AZ 85025
Phone: (602) 321-9632
Fax: (602) 321-9633
Fred Fixit, RPh

Steps to Transferring a Prescription

Use the information in the above scenario to complete the following steps.

1   Access the main menu of Visual SuperScript.

2   Click on **FILL RX'S** located on the left side of the menu screen. The *Prescription Processing* form appears.

3   From the *Prescription Processing* form, click on the **ARROW** next to **MISC** (miscellaneous) located on the bottom left corner of the form.

4   Click on **XFER OUT** (transfer out). The *Customer History: Transfer Rx Out* dialog box pops up.

5   Key in the customer name in the **CUSTOMER** data entry field. Press the **ENTER** key. The *Customer Lookup* dialog box appears. Click on the appropriate customer from the lookup list and click on **OK**.

> **LAB TIP:** Make sure that you are on the **PRESCRIPTION ON FILE** menu. Tab to mark the boxes.

6   Put a checkmark in the check box of the prescription that should be transferred to another pharmacy.

7   Click on **XFER OUT** located at the top of the dialog box. This will create a record of the transferred prescription in the patient's profile.

Note: At this time, the pharmacist or pharmacy technician at the pharmacy (depending on the state laws) will call the pharmacy to which the prescription is being transferred. Certain information is required, and **many states require a pharmacist, only, to transfer prescriptions and to accept transferred prescriptions**.

> **LAB TIP:** You may need to enter the pharmacy contact information (address and phone number) before you can transfer the prescription.

8   Print the screen by using the **PRINTSCRN** option on your keyboard. Press the **PRINTSCRN** key, open a blank Word document, right-click the blank Word document, and then select **PASTE**.

9   Complete the *Transfer Rx Out* dialog box information. Click on **TRANSFER RX** located at the bottom of the dialog box.

Putting a Prescription on File

Pre Lab Information

Often a patient may present a new prescription for filling that they may not need filled that day. They may have existing refills from a previous one already at the pharmacy or not need it for another reason. Sometimes these prescriptions medications can be "put on file" or saved for filling later.

Scenario

Mrs. Carla Watson is at the pharmacy this afternoon with two prescriptions from the dentist. One prescription is for an antibiotic and the other is for pain medication. Mrs. Watson would like to have the prescription for the antibiotic filled, but she is not sure that she needs the pain medication. "I really have no pain," she explains, "I hate to take the pain pills if I don't need them. Can you keep the prescription for pain pills in case I start having pain later this evening or tomorrow morning?"

Task

Put Mrs. Carla Watson's prescription for pain medication on file. Putting the prescription on file will electronically store the prescription for Mrs. Watson without charging her insurance company or filling the order.

R̶x̶

John Burns, DDS
123 Main Street
Brighton, MA 02135
Office: (617) 321-1123
Fax: (617) 431-5320

Patient Name: Carla Watson

Date: 7/7/2010

Address: 1010 Haverford Street, Chestnut Hill, MA 02167

Refill: 0
Rx: Tylenol c codeine #3
       i-ii po prn pain
       #10

DEA: AK6321892
State License: 2556321

Steps to Putting a Prescription on File

Use the information in the above scenario to complete the following steps.

1 Access the main menu of Visual SuperScript.

2 Click on **FILL RX'S** located on the left side of the menu screen. The *Prescription Processing* form appears.

3 From the *Prescription Processing* form, complete the patient and prescription information as you would if you were filling a new prescription. (Refer to Lab 6 for directions.)

4 After the *Prescription Processing* form is completed, click on **HOLD THIS** located at the top left corner of the form.

> **LAB TIP:** HOLD THIS is located under the *Record Rx* box.

5   Although this medication will not be filled, a label will be generated. A section of the label will be filed with the prescription hard copy for recordkeeping purposes.

6   Click on **Cus History/Refill** located on the left side of the screen. Check to ensure that the prescription has been put on file.

7   A prescription that has been put on file or "on hold" can be filled at a later date by accessing the prescription from the *Customer History/Refill Rx's* form.

LAB TIP: Note the prescription number of any medications put on hold.

Quick Challenge

You have learned how to perform many fill and refill functions. Do you know how to take the prescription off hold and return later to fill it? Take Mrs. Watson's Tylenol off hold and fill it.

Reversing a Prescription Order

Scenario

Carla Watson has decided she does not need her pain medications filled. Using the **Rx REVERSAL** directions, return the medication to stock and reverse the claim to her insurance.

Steps for Reversing a Prescription Order

Use the information in the above scenario to complete the following steps.

1   Access the main menu of Visual SuperScript.

2   Click on **FILL Rx'S** located on the left side of the menu screen. The *Prescription Processing* form appears.

3   Click on **Rx REVERSAL** button on the left side of the screen.

4   In the **Rx Reversal** box, enter in the prescription number and fill date.

5   Enter in the customer's insurance information when prompted to reverse the prescription on insurance.

6   Click **Proceed** to reverse the prescription. Continue to click **OK** or **Yes** to complete the reversal.

Extemporaneous Compounding

LAB OBJECTIVES

In this lab, you will:
- Enter new compounded drug data in the pharmacy software database.

STUDENT DIRECTIONS

Estimated completion time: 30 minutes

1. Read through the steps in the lab before performing the lab exercise.
2. After reading through the lab, perform the required steps to enter compounded drug information.
3. Practice filling a prescription using the new compounded drug information.

Pre Lab Information

A patient will often require a specific dose or dose form that is not available from the manufacturer. This circumstance is known as extemporaneous compounding or nonsterile compounding. The order resembles a recipe with ingredients individually calculated and then prepared in a lab. The following exercise demonstrates how to enter a compound prescription in the database and allows for charging all of the ingredients. Once completed, you will be able to process a compound prescription for a specific patient through a "Quick Challenge."

Steps to Enter Compound Drug Information

1 Access the main screen of Visual SuperScript.

2 Click on **DATA** from the toolbar located on the top of the screen.

3 Select **DRUGS** from the drop-down menu. A dialog box entitled *Drugs* will pop up.

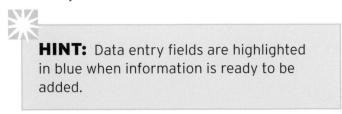

4 Click on the **NEW** icon located on the toolbar at the top of the *Drugs* dialog box. The form is now ready for you to enter information about the compounded drug.

5 Click on the **LABEL NAME** textbox field. This textbox will appear in blue when text is ready to be added.

HINT: Data entry fields are highlighted in blue when information is ready to be added.

6   Type in the name of the compounded drug that will appear on the vial label.

Enter *Judy's Antiwrinkle Cream.*

Note: Three tabbed pages appear in this form: (1) green tab—*Drug and Packaging*; (2) yellow tab—*Pricing and Stock*; and (3) pink tab—*Welfare & Misc.* Make sure you are on the **GREEN** tab to select the *Drug and Packaging* data fields.

> **LAB TIP:** Navigate through the form by using the **TAB** key.

7   Type in the **Q CODE** for the compounded drug.

Enter *Judyaw.*

Note: **QUICK CODES** (Q Codes) is a useful tool to expedite the search for drugs in your database. The **Q CODE** that you enter for your new compound should be based on the label name of the compound.

8   Key in the **ALCHEMY PRODUCT ID** for the new compounded drug.

Enter *jc2012.*

Note: The **ALCHEMY PRODUCT ID** is the lot number that was created by the pharmacy for the new compounded drug. This lot number or **ALCHEMY PRODUCT ID** must be six or less characters.

9   Click on the **ARROW** to the right of **DRUG CLASS**. The *Drug Class* combo box appears. Click on the appropriate drug class from the drop-down list. Click **OK**.

Select Rx.

10 Click on the **ARROW** to the right of **ITEM TYPE**. A list of drug item choices appears.

Click on COMPOUND from this list.

11 Indicate whether the new compound is gender-specific in the **GENDER FIELD**. Click on the **ARROW** to the right of gender to access the pick list.

Select BOTH.

12   Tab to the **BRAND/GENERIC** field. Click on the **ARROW** to the right of the field. Identify the new compound as brand or generic by clicking on the appropriate choice.

Select GENERIC.

13   Click on **DEFAULT SIG**. This new compound may frequently be prescribed with the same instructions for use. Enter the appropriate instructions for use in the text field. These default instructions may be changed when filling the prescription, if needed.

Enter *Apply to affected area.*

14   Click on the **DRUG UNIT** data field on the right side of the *Drug and Packaging* form.

15   Click on the **ARROW** to the right of **DRUG UNIT**. The *Dispensing Unit* dialog box appears. Click on the appropriate dispensing unit from the list. Click **OK**.

Select GM.

Note: *EA* means *each*; *GM* means *gram*; *ML* means *milliliter*.

16   Click on the **ARROW** to the right of **UNITS**. The *Units* dialog box appears. Click on the appropriate unit from this list. Click **OK**.

Select GM.

> **HINT:** Use the vertical scroll bar located on the right side of the *Dialog/Pop-Up* box to view the entire list.

17   Click on the **SAVE** 🖫 icon located at the top right of the toolbar. Basic information regarding the new compound has been saved to the *Drugs* form. You are now ready to add the ingredients of the new compound to the *Drugs* form. The bottom section of the *Drugs* form has three tabbed pages: (1) Yellow tab—*Manufacturing & Available NDCs*; (2) green tab—*Compounded Drug Ingredients*; and (3) blue tab—*3rd Party NDC Preferences*.

Click the GREEN tab to select COMPOUNDED DRUG INGREDIENTS.

18 Each ingredient in the new compound will be added one at a time to the grid. Click on the **NEW** ⃞ icon located at the bottom right of this *Drugs* form. Two dialog boxes pop up on the screen: *Drug Name Lookup* and *Compound Drug Ingredients*.

19 Key in the first few letters of the desired drug ingredient. Select the correct drug from the list by clicking on the drug name. Click **OK**.

**Enter *Tret* for Tretinoin 0.05% Cream.
Select the 45.0 package size for this drug.**

20 Highlight the correct medication needed, based on your prescription.

21 In the *Compound Drug Ingredients* dialog box, type in the correct quantity of drug in grams needed.

For this compound, you will need 2.5 g.

22 Click **SAVE** on the bottom of the *Compound Drug Ingredients* dialog box.

23 Continue to add each ingredient one at a time by clicking on the **NEW** ▯ icon located at the bottom right of the *Drugs* form. Review steps 19 through 22 to add each ingredient.

> **Enter *dexpa* for dexpanthenol USP powder and the quantity of *1 g*.**
>
> **Enter *water* for water for injection, 5 ml vial, and the quantity of *0.02 ml*.**

24 Once all of the ingredients are added, click the **CALCULATE PRICE** tab located at the bottom right of the toolbar. The compound is now saved.

You have completed the task of adding a new compounded drug to the pharmacy computer system and can close out of the *Drugs* dialog box.

Steps to Perform a Drug Look-Up

Perform a drug look-up to make sure the new compound has been added to the computer system correctly.

1 Click on **DATA** from the toolbar located on the top of the screen.

2 Select **DRUGS** from the drop-down menu.

3 Click on the **FIND** 🔍 icon located at the top left of the toolbar.

4 The *Drug Name Lookup* dialog box appears. Key in the label name of the new compound.

Enter *judy's* for Judy's Antiwrinkle Cream.

5 Select the correct compound from the list by clicking on the drug name. Click **OK**.

6 Read through the *Drugs* form to check for accuracy.

Print screen and save for your instructor.

7 Click on the **CLOSE** 🔲 icon on the top right of the toolbar to clear the screen.

Quick Challenge

Fill-in the medication order for the compound entered in the lab. Use the prescription on the following page for patient and prescriber information. Then you will process the prescription for the individual patient and print a label.

> **LAB TIP:** Once the compound is entered in the database, fill an Rx using the quick code you selected for the compound. This will be the *prescribed drug* for the patient.

Rx

Dr. James Furlong, II
3 Atrium Drive
Albany, NY 12205
Office: (518) 453-9080
Fax: (518) 453-9089

Patient Name: Marjorie Davidson

Address: 27 Bradord Street, Newton, MA 02456

Rx: Judy's Antiwrinkle Cream
      Tretinoin 0.05% cream, 2.5 g
      Dexpanthenol powder, 1 g
      SWFI 0.02 ml

DEA: AF9018753

Processing a New Prescription for an Insurance Patient

LAB OBJECTIVES

In this lab, you will:

- Learn how to perform necessary computer functions to enter a new prescription into a pharmacy system for the patient who has insurance.
- Learn how to process a third-party claim through online (adjudication).

STUDENT DIRECTIONS

Estimated completion time: 30 minutes

1. Read through the steps in the lab before performing the lab exercise.
2. After reading through the lab, perform the required steps to create a label and prepare the product for dispensing.
3. Complete the exercise at the end of the lab.

Pre Lab Information

Entering and verifying third-party or insurance data when processing a prescription is a major component of the community or retail setting. For instance, when a customer drops off the prescription hard copy, the customer will present a card containing pertinent information if he or she has an insurance plan that covers prescriptions. This plan may be a third-party company through an employer, Medicaid from the state, or Medicare Part D.

℞ **DAA HEALTH CARE**

Health Plan 123-45678-90
Member ID: 987654321   **Group Number:** 111222

Member: State Health Plan
  John Doe
Dependents   **Payer ID:** 12345
  Jill Doe   **Rx Plan:**
  Jack Doe   **RxBin:** 987654
                                         RxGrp: DAAHC13

State Health Plan ID: S5678_2012_95 CMS Approved 10/11
CMS_S5678 XXX

Rx Plan
RxBin: 98765
RxGrp: DAAHC13

To verify benefits, view claims, find a provider, or make inquiries, call 1-800-555-1234.

Medical claims: PO Box 33333, Nashville, TN 12345
Pharmacy claims: PO Box 44444, Nashville, TN 12345

Continued

Pre Lab Information—cont'd

After the pharmacy technician has obtained or verified all the necessary information from the customer, such as member ID number, group number, copay requirements, and coverage information, the prescription data are entered into the computer.

This lab explains the steps involved in filling a new prescription for an insurance customer. Working through the steps involved in interpreting and transcribing a prescription (Lab 6) before completing the following lab is beneficial.

Steps to Process a New Prescription for an Insurance Patient

R	**Dr. John Thompson** **81 Highland Street** **Allston, MA 02134** Office: (617) 632-4568 Fax: (617) 734-6340

Patient Name: Brian Davidson

Date: 2/17/2012

Address: 27 Bradford Street, Newton, MA

Refill: 0
Rx: Cefaclor 500 mg, qd #30
Brand Necessary

DEA: AT4278431
State License: 3445542

Use the above prescription to complete the following steps.

1 Access the main menu of Visual SuperScript.

2 Click on **FILL RX'S** located on the left side of the menu screen. The *Prescription Processing* form appears.

3 Click on the **NEW RX** icon on the top left of the *Prescription Processing* form.

Note: Prescription information such as the **RX NO.** (prescription number) and **DISPENSE DATE** are automatically generated and added to the form. You may also choose the **RX ORIGIN** from the drop-down menu if the prescription is not written.

4 Enter your initials in the *Enter Tech Init* box that appears, and click **OK**.

5 You will then be prompted to the **CUSTOMER'S LOOKUP** (highlighted in blue) text box. Type the first three letters of the last name and hit **ENTER**.

**Type *DAV* for Brian Davidson
as indicated in the sample prescription.**

6 Select the appropriate customer by double-clicking on customer name or by clicking **OK** when customer name is highlighted in blue.

Note: The customer's personal information such as **ADDRESS**, **PHONE**, and **BIRTHDATE** will be automatically added to the *Prescription Processing* form.

Note: You are automatically directed to the **DOCTOR** text box once the patient information is populated. For new prescriptions, the system will search the patient's prescription file to find the name of the prescriber of the most recently filled prescription. If found, the system will insert the prescriber's name into this field. If a different doctor has written the new prescription, you can delete the old name and enter a new one.

7 Enter *Thompson, John* into the **DOCTOR** text box as indicated on the prescription on the previous page.

8 Press the **TAB** key. You will be prompted to the **PRESCRIBED DRUG** data entry field. Key in the first three letters of the prescribed drug into the **PRESCRIBED DRUG** data entry field. Then press **ENTER**.

Enter *Cef* for Brian's Cefaclor.

9 Select the appropriate drug entitled *Drug Name Lookup* from the drop-down list by double-clicking on the drug name.

> **LAB TIP:** If a series of warning dialog boxes appear, these are known as drug utilization reviews (DURs). The patient's medication history is compared against the drug you are entering for pregnancy warnings, drug-drug and drug-food interactions, or contraindication conditions or diseases. (The warning messages should be viewed and approved by the pharmacist before dispensing the medication.)

10   After receiving approval from the *Instructor* to continue, click **Close** to move through the warnings. Click **Continue Rx** to navigate to the next step.

11   Drug information such as **NDC#** and **Manufacturer** will appear under **Available Drug Choice**. Choose the generic substitution unless the doctor has specified, "dispense as written" (DAW).

12   Next, you will be prompted to the **Refills Ordered** data entry field. Key in the appropriate number of refills.

13   Press the **Tab** key. You will be prompted to enter the prescribed quantity. Key in the appropriate quantity in the **Prescribed Quantity** data entry field.

14   Press the **Tab** key until you reach the **DAW** text box. Choose the correct **DAW** code by clicking on the **Arrow** on the right side of the **DAW** data entry field. Click on the correct **DAW** code from the pick list.

Note: When filling a prescription, knowing the correct **DAW** code to be assigned to a prescription is necessary for reimbursement. For this to be accomplished, distinguish between the brand name and the generic name of the medication. Although the prescriber may write the brand name of a drug on a patient's prescription, it may not necessarily mean that the brand-name drug must be dispensed. If the prescriber indicates **DAW** or "brand name medically necessary" on the patient's prescription for a brand-name drug, then the brand-name drug rather than the generic alternative MUST be dispensed. This situation, for example, would be a **DAW** code 1. The failure to use the proper **DAW** codes may result in improper third-party reimbursement to the pharmacy. Seven **DAW** codes are used in the pharmacy practice:

DAW 0—Physician has approved the dispensing of a generic medication.

DAW 1—Physician requests that the brand-name drug be dispensed.

DAW 2—Physician has approved the dispensing of a generic drug, but the patient has requested that the brand-name drug be dispensed.

DAW 3—Pharmacist dispenses the drug as written.

DAW 4—No generics are available in the store.

DAW 5—Brand-name drug is dispensed but priced as a generic drug.

DAW 6—RPh doctor call is attempted.

15   Press the **Tab** key. Key in the patient abbreviated directions in the **Sig** text box.

Key in T1T QD PO as the shortcut abbreviation sig
for Brian Davidson.

Note: What appears in the blue **SIG IN ENGLISH** space is what will appear on the label. If an error is made when typing in the sig, backspace to delete the error and retype the correct information.

16 Press the **TAB** key. You will be prompted to enter **PRESCRIBED DAYS SUPPLY**. Key in the appropriate days supply in the **PRESCRIBED DAYS SUPPLY** data entry field.

ENTER *30* for Brian Davidson's days supply.

Note: Days supply involves calculating the number of days that a particular prescription will last. All third-party payers require this information. The failure to provide days supply information properly may result in the pharmacy losing money. To calculate the days supply a prescription will last, use the following formula:

$$\text{Days supply} = \frac{\text{Total quantity dispensed}}{\text{Total quantity taken per day}}$$

The days supply is the number of days a medication will last for one filling. Days supply does not take into account refills. The majority of the third-party payers will reimburse a pharmacy for a 30-day supply of medication.

Note: You may tab back to the **RX NOTES** section and add any notes that apply. Most states require patients to receive the opportunity for medication counseling. The **RX NOTES** section is a good spot to document "offered counseling, but patient refused counseling" or other similar important information.

17 Press the **ENTER** key. You are now prompted to save the prescription information. Click the **SAVE** 💾 icon.

> **HINT:** Make sure you save using the **SAVE** button to the right. (Save this Rx in the System Memory.) Visual SuperScript will default to the **SAVE** button on the left, which will save the entry and automatically move you to a new prescription for the same customer. If you use the **SAVE** button on the left and the screen goes blank, then you can click the **BACK** button to reclaim the Rx and print the label.

18 Click on **LABEL** on the left of the screen to complete adjudication and **PRINT** 🖨 .

19 Prepare the medication for dispensing, including labeling the product. Affix the second label to the back of the original prescription.

Note: The label has two amounts: (1) price and (2) copay. These amounts reflect the amount the insurance allows for the drug (price) and the amount the customer must pay as his or her part (copay).

Exercise

Enter prescriptions and prepare products for dispensing using the assigned prescriptions found in Appendix B. Leave the stock bottle, original prescription, and prepared product for a pharmacist final check. Remember to affix the second label on the back of the original prescription in your book.

The customer's personal information such as **ADDRESS**, **PHONE**, and **BIRTHDATE** will automatically be added to the *Prescription Processing* form, but you will need to verify the insurance coverage by reviewing the card information and making any changes as required.

R̫x

Dr. John Thompson
81 Highland Street
Allston, MA 02134
Office: (617) 632-4568
Fax: (617) 734-6340

Patient Name: Cynthia Franks

Date: 2/17/2012

Address: 123 Long Avenue, Brighton, MA

Refill: 5
Rx: Coumadin 5 mg, qd #30
Brand Necessary

DEA: AT4278431
State License: 3445542

Note: Practice using the abbreviation shortcuts found in Appendix A to make the process quicker. All drug community software programs use these abbreviations to save time. Some prescriptions may require adding new patient information, new prescriber information, or adding a new drug to the database. You may review Section 1 for these procedures.

Blister Packing: Batch Filling for a Nursing Home

LAB OBJECTIVES

In this lab, you will:

- Learn how to refill a group of prescriptions ordered for a nursing home.
- Learn how to prepare the medications using blister packing.
- Learn how to prepare a report for a nursing home.

STUDENT DIRECTIONS

Estimated completion time: 1 hour

1. Read through the steps in the lab before performing the lab exercise.
2. After reading through the lab, perform the required steps to complete the tasks in each scenario.
3. Answer the questions at the end of the lab..

Pre Lab Information

Nursing homes and long-term care facilities often contract with local pharmacies to prepare their residents' monthly medications. This is done using cards or containers that have individual pockets designed to hold dosages. For example, a person's morning and nightly medications can be packed in different pockets, similar to a daily pillbox. This approach allows for routine dose changes and the return of medications that often occur in this population.

Scenario

Mrs. Davis at the Coolidge Corner Nursing Home called to ask for some of the residents' refills.

Beaty, Okla: simvastatin, 20 mg, and Lopressor, 100 mg

Busch, Jane: Lipitor, 20 mg, and Coumadin, 10 mg

Busch, John: Lipitor, 20 mg, and Coumadin, 1 mg

Ellis, Floyd: omeprazole

Fletcher, Irene: glipizide, atenolol, and metformin

Hatcher, Ernest: Risperdal and Motrin

Horton, Mary E: ferrous sulfate

Richey, Thelma: hydrochlorothiazide (HCTZ)

Task

You must first look up the patients and find their prescription numbers. Look for the most current prescriptions (dates). You will refill the prescriptions, prepare them using the blister packing method, and prepare a report for the residents medications for billing.

Steps to Prepare a Batch Refill

Use the above information box to complete the following steps for each customer.

1 Access the main menu of Visual SuperScript.

2 Click on **FILL RX'S** located on the left side of the menu screen. The *Prescription Processing* form appears.

3 From the *Prescription Processing* form, click on the **ARROW** next to the **REFILL RX'S** menu on the left of the form to access the expanded **REFILL RX'S** menu.

4 Click on **CUS HISTORY/REFILL**.

5 Key the first customer name into the **CUSTOMER** data entry field of the *Customer History: Refill Rx's* dialog box. Press the **ENTER** key. The *Customer Lookup* dialog box appears. Click on the correct customer from the list in the *Customer Lookup* dialog box. Click on **OK**.

Enter customer name *Beaty, Okla.*

6 Select the tab titled **PRESCRIPTIONS ON FILE**. Put a checkmark in the checkbox of the first prescription that needs to be refilled.

Check the box for *simvastatin* and *lopressor*.

7 Click on **REFILL RX** located at the top of the dialog box.

Customer History: Refill Rx's											

Customer: BEATY, OKLA Address: 85 CHERRY STREET Phone: (617) 532-2672 Birthdate: 04/01/1922 [Refill Rx] [Cancel] User Interface: ● Basic ○ Advance

Prescriptions on File= 7 , # Selected for Refills= 1   Refill History

R	Rx #	Pres Date ↑	Prescribed Drug	Quantity	Days Supply	Rem. Qty	Rem. Days	Last Fill Date	Last Disp. Qty	Doctor
☐	387579	10/07/2009	KEFLEX 500 MG PULVULE	62.000	31	312.000		04/30/2009	60.000	SCHOULTIES, JOHN
☑	387464	05/27/2009	SIMVASTATIN 20 MG TABLET	30.000	30	120.000		05/27/2009	30.000	SCHOULTIES, JOHN
☐	387454	05/14/2009	TOPAMAX 100 MG TABLET	30.000	30	60.000		05/14/2009	30.000	SCHOULTIES, JOHN
☐	387453	05/14/2009	LOPRESSOR 100 MG TABLET	2.000	1	2.000		05/14/2009	2.000	SCHOULTIES, JOHN
☐	387370	03/31/2009	KEFLEX 500 MG PULVULE	62.000	31	0.000		03/31/2009	60.000	SCHOULTIES, JOHN
☐	387080	05/09/2007	KEFLEX 500 MG PULVULE	62.000	31	252.000		06/01/2007	60.000	SCHOULTIES, JOHN
☐	386725	03/08/2005	KEFLEX 500 MG PULVULE	28.000	14	0.000		03/08/2005	28.000	SCHOULTIES, JOHN

Hot Keys	M= Menu	A= Show All D= Show Selected Drug Only R= Selected for Refills H= Refill History F= Fill Rx
		S= Sort On Prescribed / Dispensed Date E= Edit Prescription I= Inactivate Rx T= Transfer Rx Out

[Show All]   [Selected Drug]   [Selected For Refills]   [Drug] [_____]

> **LAB TIP:** If the prescription has *not* expired and refills remain, the *Prescription Processing* form is updated with the refill information. If the prescription has expired, the **CANNOT REFILL, SELECT COPY OPTIONS** screen will appear. Complete the process of requesting refill authorization (Lab 7) to refill each prescription.

8 The *Prescription Processing* form now returns to the screen. The medication checked in the box will be ready to process. Click on **LABEL** located at the top left of the form, which will prompt the software to adjudication and print a label.

9 Continue with each medication requested by following the previous steps.

Preparing the Report

Once the medications are refilled according to the list provided by the nursing home, a report can be generated for billing and verifying each transaction.

Steps to Prepare a Batch Refill Report

1   Access the main screen of Visual SuperScript.

2   Click on **REPORTS** from the menu toolbar located at the top of the screen.

3   Select **CUSTOMER REPORTS** from the drop-down menu. Then select **CUSTOMER HISTORY** from the expanded menu.

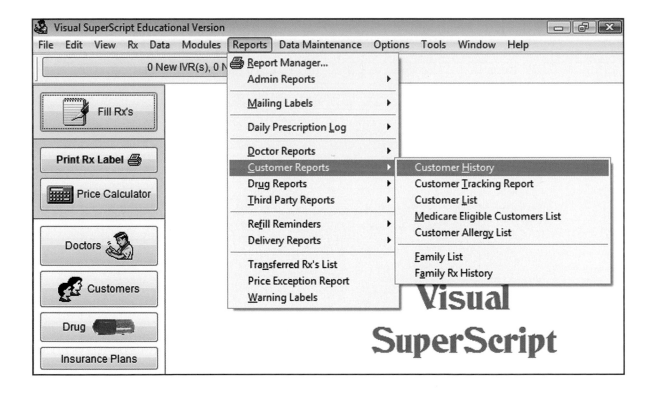

4   The *Customer History* dialog box appears. Notice that the insertion point is in the first data entry field, **DATE FROM**. Key in the date that the *Customer History Report* should start.

Key in today's date.

5 Key in the date that the *Customer History Report* should end in the **To** data entry field.

Key in today's date.

> **LAB TIP:** Deleting the default date that appears in the data entry field is not necessary. The date that is keyed in will replace the existing default date.

6 The **SHOW** field will designate if the report should be generated to show the **COPAY** amount for the medications or the actual **PRICE** of the medications. Click on the appropriate choice.

Select Copay.

7 The **FORMAT** field will designate if the report should be generated in an **INSURANCE** format or a **NHOME** (nursing home) format.

**Select NHOME format
since the patient is a resident of a nursing home.**

8 Select the **NEW PAGE FOR EACH CUSTOMER** field if individual pages are desired.

9 The **FOR** data field offers several different choices in generating the *Customer History Report*. Select one of the five choices in which the *Customer History Report* will be generated. Click on the appropriate choice.

Select Individual Customer.

10 The customer name entry field will ask for the customer name or the name of the insurance plan. The required information depends on the selection made in step 9.

Key in *Beaty, Okla.*

> **LAB TIP:** Enter the first three letters of the patient's last name, and hit **ENTER** to search for the customer in the customer lookup field.

11   Click on **PREVIEW** located the bottom of the *Customer History* dialog box. The selected *Customer History Report* will open and appear on the screen.

12   Click on the **PRINT REPORT** icon located at the top right of the *Report Designer* toolbar.

13   Click on the **CLOSE PREVIEW** icon located at the top right of the *Report Designer* toolbar. The report is closed out and the *Customer History* dialog box returns.

14   Follow these steps to create a report for each customer on your list.

INSTITUTIONAL PHARMACY PRACTICE

Entering New Intravenous Orders

LAB OBJECTIVES

In this lab, you will:

- Interpret a hospital intravenous (IV) order.
- Enter a new IV order from an institutional order.

STUDENT DIRECTIONS

Estimated completion time: 30 minutes

1. Read through the steps in the lab before performing the lab exercise.
2. After reading through the lab, perform the required steps to enter compounded drug information.
3. Practice filling a prescription using the new compounded drug information.

Pre Lab Information

Institutional pharmacy orders differ from prescriptions because the patient is considered *inpatient*, and any instructions related to patient care while he or she is staying in the health care facility is written on the order sheet. Other information such as laboratory work, diet, routine vital signs, and tests are included on the same order, and a technician must be able to pull out the medications. When entering a new IV order, additives and a base fluid will be listed. These components must be added individually and charged accordingly.

Steps to Enter a New Intravenous Order

1   Check your printer settings.

    a   Go to **OPTIONS** on the top tool bar of Visual SuperScript.

    b   Choose **Rx LABEL OPTIONS**.

    c   Change *Label Type* to **TPN**.

    d   *WorkFlow Label* can remain as the default—**LM32**.

    e   Click **OK** on the bottom right of window.

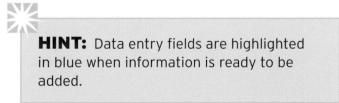

2   Access the main screen of Visual SuperScript.

3   Click on **DATA** from the toolbar located on the top of the screen.

4   Select **DRUGS** from the drop-down menu. A dialog box entitled *Drugs* will pop up.

5   Click on the **NEW** ☐ icon located on the toolbar at the top of the *Drugs* dialog box. The form is now ready for you to enter information about the compounded drug.

6   Click on the **LABEL NAME** textbox field.

> **HINT:** Data entry fields are highlighted in blue when information is ready to be added.

7   Type in the name of the compounded IV order that will appear on the
     IV label.

Enter *LR with 25 mEq Mag Sulfate*.

Note: Three tabbed pages are provided on this form: (1) green tab—*Drug
     and Packaging; (2) yellow tab—*Pricing and Stock*; and (3) pink
     tab—*Welfare & Misc*. Make sure you are on the **Green** tab to
     select the *Drug and Packaging* data fields.

> **LAB TIP:** Navigate through the form by using
> the tab key.

8   Type in the **Q Code** for the compounded drug.

Enter *LR25MAG*.

Note: Quick Codes (Q Codes) is a useful tool to expedite the search for
     drugs in your database. The **Q Code** that you enter for your new
     compound should be based on the label name of the compound.

9   Click on the **Arrow** to the right of **Drug Class**. The *Drug Class* combo
     box appears. Click on the appropriate drug class from the drop-down
     list. Click **OK**.

Select Rx.

10   Click on the **Arrow** to the right of **Item Type**. A list of drug item
     choices appears.

Click on Compound from this list.

11   Indicate whether the new compound is gender-specific in the **Gender
     Field**. Click on the **Arrow** to the right of gender to access the pick list.

Select Both.

12   Tab to the **Brand/Generic** field. Click on the **Arrow** to the right of
     the field. Identify the new compound as brand or generic by clicking on
     the appropriate choice.

Select Generic.

13 Click on the **ARROW** to the right of **DRUG UNIT**. The *Dispensing Unit* dialog box appears. Click on the appropriate dispensing unit from the list. Click **OK**.

Select ML.

Note: *EA* means *each*; *GM* means *gram*; *ML* means *milliliter*.

14 Click on the **ARROW** to the right of **UNITS**. The *Units* dialog box appears. Click on the appropriate unit from this list. Click **OK**.

Select ML.

15 Tab to the **PACKAGE SIZE** field.

Enter *1000 ml* for the package size.

16 Tab to **DAYS TO EXPIRE**.

Enter *1 day*.

17 Tab to **DEFAULT SIG**. This new compound may frequently be prescribed with the same instructions for use. Enter the appropriate instructions for use in the text field. These default instructions may be changed when filling the prescription, if needed.

Enter *infuse at 125 ml/hr*.

Note: These default instructions may be changed when filling the prescription, if needed.

> **HINT:** Use the vertical scroll bar located on the right side of the dialog/pop-up box to view the entire list.

18 Click on the **SAVE** 🖫 icon located at the top right of the toolbar. Basic information regarding the new compound has been saved to the *Drugs* form. You are now ready to add the ingredients of the new compound to the *Drugs* form. The bottom section of the *Drugs* form has three tabbed pages: (1) Yellow tab—*Manufacturing & Available NDCs*; (2) green tab—*Compounded Drug Ingredients*; and (3) blue tab—*Third Party NDC Preferences*.

Click the GREEN tab to select COMPOUNDED DRUG INGREDIENTS.

19 Each additive and amount needed in the new compound will be added one at a time to the grid. Click on the **NEW** ☐ icon located at the bottom right of this *Drugs* form. Two dialog boxes pop up on the screen: *Drug Name Lookup* and *Compound Drug Ingredients*.

20 Key in the first few letters of the desired drug ingredient. Select the correct drug from the list by clicking on the drug name. Click **OK**.

> **Enter *LAC* for lactated Ringers 500 ml (base fluid).**

21 Click on the **SAVE** button on the bottom of the *Compound Drug Ingredients* dialog box.

22 Continue to add each ingredient one at a time by clicking on the **NEW** ☐ icon located at the bottom right of this *Drugs* form. Review steps 19 through 21 to add each ingredient.

> **Enter *Mag* for magnesium sulfate**
> **50% vial additive ingredient (20.0 pkg size).**

Note: You must recalculate the amount needed to be drawn up and choose the correct package size. In this example, magnesium sulfate comes as 4 meg, so 20 mEq would require 6.25 ml to be drawn up.

23 Click on the **CLOSE** ⏏ icon located at the top right of the toolbar. You have completed the task of adding a new IV order to the pharmacy computer system!

24 Perform a drug look-up to make sure the new compound has been added to the computer system correctly.

25 Click on **DATA** from the toolbar located on the top of the screen.

26 Select **DRUGS** from the drop-down menu.

27 Click on the **FIND** 🔍 icon located at the top left of the toolbar.

28 The *Drug Name Lookup* dialog box appears. Key in the label name of the new compound.

> **Enter *LR* to search for lactated Ringers**
> **with 25 mEq Mag sulfate**
> **or use the quick code you selected—LR25MAG.**

29   Select the correct compound from the list by clicking on the drug name. Click **OK**.

30   Read through the *Drugs* form to check for accuracy. Click on the **CLOSE** ▯◄ icon on the top right of the toolbar to clear the screen.

Drugs

Q M ▦ Y a..z ⎙   ⏮ ◀ ▶ ⏭   ☐ ▤ ▨ ✕ ✂ ▦ 🖫 ↺ ▯◄

ADD Drug By NDC	FDB Standard Name	Label Name
		LR WITH 25 MEQ KCL

Drug and Packaging	Pricing and Stock	Welfare & Misc

Drug and Class Type   ## Packaging

Quick Code	LR25KCL	Form	
Alchemy Product ID		Strength	
		Drug Unit	ML ⬇
Drug Class	RX ⬇	Units	ML ⬇
Item Type	Compound ▾	Package Size	
Gender	BOTH ▾		
Brand/Generic	Generic ▾	Days to Expire	365
		Max Dose	

Default NDC	00000-0000-00	☐ No Default NDC	Default Quantity	
Default Sig	125 ML/HR		Default Day Supply	

Equivalent Drug		⬇

Manufacturer & Available NDCs	Compound Drug Ingredients	3rd Party NDC Preferences

Drug Name	Drug NDC	Quantity	Cost Basis	Cost	
LACTATED RINGERS INJECTION	00409-7953-03		AWP ▾		
MAGNESIUM SULFATE 50% VIAL	00409-2168-03		AWP ▾		

Route of Admin 00
Dosage Form

Cost Basis
AWP ▾

Calculate Price

☐ ✕

Quick Challenge

Fill in the intravenous (IV) order for the patient below. Make sure that the compound in the medication order has been properly added to the drug database. Print a label for the patient when all the information is entered.

Patient Name Myrtle York	Diet REG	Weight 134 lb	Height 64
Room Number 420	Diagnosis		
Hospital Number 123334	R/O sepsis, dehydration		
Attending Physician Stephen Hardy	Drug Allergies NKDA		

DATE	TIME		
5/19	0615	Admit to CCU	
		LR 1 liter with 25 mEq Magnesium sulfate @ 125ml/hr	
		X 1 bag	
		——— v/o K Davis, RN. 5/19 0620	

> **LAB TIP:** Once the compound is entered in the database, fill an Rx using the quick code you selected for the compound. This will be the *Prescribed Drug* for the patient.

Additional Exercises

1   Fill the medication orders in Appendix D. You will need to perform a drug look-up to ensure the new compound has been added to the computer system correctly. If not, you will need to enter the compound as shown in this lab first. Then you will process the prescription for the individual patient and print a label.

2   Using the IV orders found in Appendix D, calculate the milliliters needed to prepare the IVs found on the hospital orders. Remember to use any approved reference for storage, dilution, and any special instructions needed for preparation. Once you have prepared a label using the steps in this lab, prepare the IV order using aseptic technique.

> **LAB TIP:** Remember to ensure that the patient profile is up-to-date when filling an institutional order.

Entering Total Parenteral Nutrition Orders

Pre Lab Information

Pharmacy personnel prepare individualized TPNs for patients who are unable to eat or receive adequate nutrition. TPN is a solution commonly made up of three base components: glucose, fats, and amino acids. Electrolytes, as well as other medications, will be added to the base TPN solution according to physician orders. TPN solutions are infused or administered to the patient through a vein. A patient may need a TPN for a variety of reasons—malnourishment because of illness, diseased state of the digestive system, or surgical procedures performed on the digestive system.

Steps to Enter a Total Parenteral Nutrition Order

1 Check your printer settings.
   a Go to **OPTIONS** on the top tool bar of Visual SuperScript.
   b Choose **RX LABEL OPTIONS**.
   c Change *Label Type* to **TPN**.
   d *WorkFlow Label* can remain as the default—**LM32**.
   e Click **OK** on the bottom right of window.

2 Access the main screen of Visual SuperScript.

3 Click on **DATA** from the toolbar located on the top of the screen.

4 Select **DRUGS** from the drop-down menu. A dialog box entitled *Drugs* will pop up.

5 Click on the **NEW** 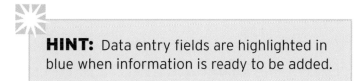 icon located on the toolbar at the top of the *Drugs* dialog box. The form is now ready for you to enter information about the TPN solution.

6 Click on the **LABEL NAME** textbox field.

> **HINT:** Data entry fields are highlighted in blue when information is ready to be added.

7 Type in the name of the compounded intravenous (IV) order that will appear on the IV label.

Enter *TPN Base.*

Note: Three tabbed pages are provided on this form: (1) green tab—*Drug and Packaging*; (2) yellow tab—*Pricing and Stock*; and (3) pink tab—*Welfare & Misc.* Make sure you are on the **GREEN** tab to select the *Drug and Packaging* data fields.

> **LAB TIP:** Navigate through the form by using the tab key.

8 Type in the **Q CODE** for the compounded drug.

Enter *TPN.*

Note: QUICK CODES (Q Codes) is a useful tool to expedite the search for drugs in your database. The **Q CODE** that you enter for your new compound should be based on the label name of the compound.

9 Click on the **Arrow** to the right of **Drug Class**. The *Drug Class* combo box appears. Click on the appropriate drug class from the drop-down list. Click **OK**.

Select Rx.

10 Click on the **Arrow** to the right of **Item Type**. A list of drug item choices appears.

Click on Compound from this list.

11 Indicate whether the new compound is gender-specific in the **Gender Field**. Click on the **Arrow** to the right of gender to access the pick list.

Select Both.

12 Tab to the **Brand/Generic** field. Click on the **Arrow** to the right of the field. Identify the new compound as brand or generic by clicking on the appropriate choice.

Select Generic.

13 Click on **Form** on the right side of the *Drug and Packaging* form. Type in the abbreviated text for IV solution.

Enter *IV solute*.

14 Click on the **Arrow** to the right of **Drug Unit**. The *Dispensing Unit* dialog box appears. Click on the appropriate dispensing unit from the list. Click **OK**.

Select ML.

Note: *EA* means *each*; *GM* means *gram*; *ML* means *milliliter*.

15 Click on the **Arrow** to the right of **Units**. The *Units* dialog box appears. Click on the appropriate unit from this list. Click **OK**.

Select ML.

16 Tab to the **Package Size** field.

Enter *1000 ml* for package size.

Note: This unit indicates a final container bag of 1000 ml or 1 L.

17 Tab to **Default Sig**. TPNs may be frequently prescribed with the same infusion rate.

Enter *infuse at 83 mL/hr*.

Note: These default instructions may be changed when filling the prescription, if needed.

18 Click on the **SAVE** 🖫 icon located at the top right of the toolbar.

> **HINT:** Use the vertical scroll bar located on the right side of the dialog/pop-up box to view the entire list.

19 Basic information regarding the new TPN base solution has been saved to the *Drugs* form. You are now ready to add the ingredients of the base TPN to the *Drugs* form. The bottom section of the *Drugs* form has three tabbed pages: (1) Yellow tab—*Manufacturing & Available NDCs*; (2) green tab—*Compounded Drug Ingredients*; and (3) blue tab—*Third Party NDC Preferences*.

Click the GREEN tab to select COMPOUNDED DRUG INGREDIENTS.

20 Each ingredient in the new compound will be added one at a time to the grid. Click on the **NEW** 🗋 icon located at the bottom right of this *Drugs* form. Two dialog boxes pop up on the screen: *Drug Name Lookup* and *Compound Drug Ingredients*.

21 Key in the first few letters of Travasol.

Enter *Trav*.
**Select *Travasol 10% IV solution—package size 500 mL*
from the list by clicking on the drug name.
Click OK.**

22 The *Compound Drug Ingredients* dialog box remains on the screen. Tab to **QUANTITY** field.

Enter *500* (for 500 ml).

Note: This number indicates the amount of Travasol added to the base TPN solution: 500 ml.

23 Click on the **SAVE** button on the bottom of the *Compound Drug Ingredients* dialog box.

24 Continue to add each ingredient in the base TPN solution one at a time by clicking on the **NEW** 🗋 icon located at the bottom right of this *Drugs* form. Review steps 21 through 23 to add each ingredient.

Enter *Dextrose 70% (D$_{70}$W)—package size 500 ml*.
Enter *350 mL* for QUANTITY.
Enter *Liposyn II 10% fat emulsion—package size 500 ml*.
Enter *100 mL* for QUANTITY.

25 Click the **CALCULATE PRICE** button at the bottom of the page. You will see an "information saved" message on the right of the screen. You have completed the task of adding a base TPN solution to the pharmacy computer system! Click on the **CLOSE** 📲 icon located at the top right of the toolbar.

24 Perform a drug look-up to make sure the new compound has been added to the computer system correctly.

25 Click on **DATA** from the toolbar located on the top of the screen.

26 Select **DRUGS** from the drop-down menu.

27   Click on the **FIND** 🔍 icon located at the top left of the toolbar.

28   The *Drug Name Lookup* dialog box appears.

Enter *TPN base.*

Drug Name Lookup						
Name TPN				☐ Show Hidden Drugs		
Drug	Pkg. Size	QuickCode	Form	Strength	Brand/Gen	▲
TPN BASE	1000.000	TPN	IV SOLUT		Generic	
						▼
				OK	Cancel	

29   Click on **TPN BASE** from the list. Click **OK**.

30   Read through the *Drugs* form to check for accuracy. Click on the **CLOSE** 🚪 icon on the top right of the toolbar to clear the screen.

Steps to Add Electrolytes

Add electrolytes to the TPN base solution, which will be determined by the order and the amounts previously calculated.

1   Click on the **DRUG** icon located on the toolbar on the left side of the main screen.

2   A dialog box entitled *Drugs* will pop up.

3   Click on the **FIND** 🔍 icon located at the top left of the toolbar.

4   The *Drug Name Lookup* dialog box appears.

Enter *TPN base.*

5   Click on **TPN BASE** from the list. Click **OK**.

> **Note:** You will see ingredients found in this base solution. Now add the electrolytes one at a time and in order.

6 Click on and select the **GREEN** tab on the bottom of the page: *Compound Drug Ingredients*.

7 Click on the **NEW** 🗋 icon located at the bottom right of this *Drugs* form. Two dialog boxes pop up on the screen: *Drug Name Lookup* and *Compound Drug Ingredients*.

8 Key in the first few letters of the first electrolyte ordered.

Enter *Pot* for potassium chloride, and choose *20 ml vial with 2 mEq/ml*.

Enter the *quantity of milliliters needed*, based on your calculations (7.5 ml needed for this order).

Click on SAVE on the bottom of this drop-down box.

LAB TIP: If other electrolytes need to be added, remember to add them one at a time by following steps 21 through 23.

9 Once all of the ingredients are added and calculations are double checked, click **CALCULATE PRICE** on the bottom of this dialog box.

10 Click the **CLOSE** 🔳 icon located at the top right of the toolbar. You have completed the task of editing computerized data to add electrolytes and other ingredients to the base TPN solution.

Quick Challenge

Fill the TPN order for the patient below. Make sure that the compound in the medication order has been properly added to the drug database. Print a label for the patient when all the information is added.

HT: **139.7** cm   WT: **51.8** kg   Patient: **Erma Campbell BD: 10/3/24**

Adult *Total* Parenteral Nutrition Order Form (Central Line Only)

Date 2/2	Is central line access in place? [ ]No [x] Yes
Time 0930	
	Type **grosshong** Date placed **2/1/2012**

Please note: Prescribers must make selections in section 1-6 of form

1. Base Formula (Check one)	2. Infusion Schedule
[ ] Standard Base: dextrose 20% and amino acids (AA) 4.25% (D40W mL and AA 8.5% 500 mL)	Rate: **83mL/hour**
[x] Individual base: Dextrose % and AA %:	**Cycling Schedule (home TPN only)**
(final concentration)	Cycle mL fluid over hours
OR	
Dextrose **70%** **400mL**	Begin at _____
AA **10%** **500mL**	

3. Standard Electrolytes/Additives	OR Specify Individualized Electrolytes/Additives		
Check here [ ]	Specify amount of electrolyte	Check all the apply	
NaCl 40 mEq / L	NaCl **30** **mEq / L**	[x] Adult MVI 5 mLs / day	
NaAc 20 mEq / L	NaAc mEq / L	[x] MTE – 5 5 mLs / day	
KCl 20 mEq / L	NaPhos mEq / L	[ ] Regular Human Insulin	
Kphos 22 mEq / L	KCl **15** mEq / L	units / Liter	
CaGlu 4.7 mEq / L	KAc mEq / L	[ ] Vitamin C 500 mg / day	
MagSO4 8 mEq / L	Kphos mEq / L	[ ] H 2 antagonist mg / day	
Adult MVI 10 mLs / day	CaGlu mEq / L	drug	
MTE-5 3 mLs / day	Mag SO4 mEq / L	[ ] Other additives	
DO NOT USE IN RENAL DYSFUNCTION!	Maximum Phosphate (Na phos _____		
	40 mEq / L or K phos 44 mEq / L _____		
	and maximum clearance 10 mEq / L		

4. Lipids (Check one)	5. Blood Glucose monitoring orders
Infuse lipids over 12 hours IV	Blood glucose monitoring every **12** hours with
[ ] 20% 250 mL every Tuesday/Thursday	sliding scale regular human insulin.
[ ] 20% 250 mL every day	Route (Circle one) **SQ** IV
[ ] 20% 250 mL every other day	**Sliding Scale** (Check one)
[x] Other schedule	[x] Sliding scale per T and T protocol
Liposyn 10% 100mls _____	[ ] Individualized sliding scale (write below)

Additional Orders (All patients)	6. Routine Laboratory Orders (Check all that apply)
1. Consult Nutrition Support Team.	[ ] BMP, Mg, Phos every AM X 3 days then every Monday & Thursday
2. CMP, Mg, Phos, triglyceride, prealbumin in the AM.	[ ] Prealbumin every Monday
3. Weigh patient daily.	[ ] Metabolic study per RT (University only)
4. Strict I/O & document in chart.	[ ] 24 hour UUN and creatinine clearance
5. Keep TPN line inviolate.	
6. If TPN interrupted for any reason, hang D10W@ current TPN rate.	

Physician Signature

> **LAB TIP:** Once the compound is entered in the database, fill an Rx using the quick code you selected for the compound. This will be the prescribed drug for the patient.

Additional Exercises

1 Fill the medication orders in Appendix F. You will need to perform a drug look-up to make sure the new TPN has been correctly added to the computer system. If not, you will need to enter the TPN as shown in this lab first. Then you will process the prescription for the individual patient and print a label.

2 Using one of the TPN orders found in Appendix F, calculate the amount of grams and milliliters needed for the order and complete and print a TPN label. Show your work.

Entering New Chemotherapy Intravenous Orders

LAB OBJECTIVES

In this lab, you will:

- Interpret a hospital chemotherapy intravenous (IV) order.
- Enter a new chemotherapy IV order from an institutional order.

STUDENT DIRECTIONS

Estimated completion time: 30 minutes

1. Read through the steps in the lab before performing the lab exercise.
2. After reading through the lab, perform the required steps to enter compounded drug information.
3. Practice filling a prescription using the new compounded drug information.

Pre Lab Information

Chemotherapy medications are often infused in a hospital, but they can also be given in an outpatient setting such as a clinic or physician's office. The orders differ from prescriptions because the dosage is determined on the patient's weight in kilograms and is most often written as micrograms per kilograms (mcg/kg). If the patient's order is written during a hospital stay, then additional instructions related to the patient's care while he or she is staying is written on the same order sheet. Other information such as laboratory work, diet, routine vital signs, and tests are included on the same order, and a technician must be able to pull out the medications. When entering a new chemotherapy IV order, a chemotherapy drug will be added to an IV solution. These components must be added individually and charged accordingly.

Physician Order

Room: 422

Patient Name: Fredonna Clift

DOB: 7/20/1921

Prescribing physician's name: J. Schoulties

Rx: Etoposide 200 mg/NS 500 ml
                   Infuse over 60 minutes x 1 bag

                   No refills

Steps to Enter a Chemotherapy Intravenous Order

1 Check your printer settings.
   a Go to **OPTIONS** on the top tool bar of Visual SuperScript.
   b Choose **RX LABEL OPTIONS**.
   c Change *Label Type* to **TPN**.
   d *WorkFlow Label* can remain as the default—**LM32**.
   e Click **OK** on the bottom right of window.

2 Access the main screen of Visual SuperScript.

3 Click on **DATA** from the toolbar located on the top of the screen.

4 Select **DRUGS** from the drop-down menu. A dialog box entitled *Drugs* will pop up.

5 Click on the **NEW** ▯ icon located on the toolbar at the top of the *Drugs* dialog box. The form is now ready for you to enter information about the TPN solution.

6 Click on the **LABEL NAME** textbox field.

> **HINT:** Data entry fields are highlighted in blue when information is ready to be added.

7   Type in the name of the compounded IV order that will appear on the IV label.

Enter *Etoposide 200 mg/NS 500 ml.*

Note: Three tabbed pages are provided on this form: (1) green tab—*Drug and Packaging*; (2) yellow tab—*Pricing and Stock*; and (3) pink tab—*Welfare & Misc.* Make sure you are on the **GREEN** tab to select the *Drug and Packaging* data fields.

> **LAB TIP:** Navigate through the form by using the tab key.

8   Type in the **Q CODE** for the compounded drug.

Enter *ETO200IV.*

Note: **QUICK CODES** (Q Codes) is a useful tool to expedite the search for drugs in your database. The **Q CODE** that you enter for your new compound should be based on the label name of the compound.

9   Click on the **ARROW** to the right of **DRUG CLASS**. The *Drug Class* combo box appears. Click on the appropriate drug class from the drop-down list. Click **OK**.

Select *Rx.*

10   Click on the **ARROW** to the right of **ITEM TYPE**. A list of drug item choices appears.

Click on COMPOUND from this list.

11   Indicate whether the new compound is gender-specific in the **GENDER FIELD**. Click on the **ARROW** to the right of gender to access the pick list.

Select BOTH.

12   Tab to the **BRAND/GENERIC** field. Click on the **ARROW** to the right of the field. Identify the new compound as brand or generic by clicking on the appropriate choice.

Select GENERIC.

13   Click on **FORM** data field on the right side of the screen.

Enter *IV solute*.

14   Click on the **ARROW** to the right of **DRUG UNIT**. The *Dispensing Unit* dialog box appears. Click on the appropriate dispensing unit from the list. Click **OK**.

Select ML.

Note: *EA* means *each*; *GM* means *gram*; *ML* means *milliliter*.

15 Click on the **ARROW** to the right of **UNITS**. The *Units* dialog box appears. Click on the appropriate unit from this list. Click **OK**.

Select ML.

16 Tab to the **PACKAGE SIZE** field.

Enter *500 ml* for package size.

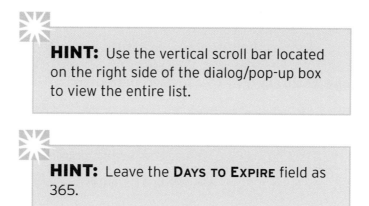

HINT: Use the vertical scroll bar located on the right side of the dialog/pop-up box to view the entire list.

HINT: Leave the **DAYS TO EXPIRE** field as 365.

17 Tab to **DEFAULT SIG**. This new compound may be frequently prescribed with the same instructions for use. Enter the appropriate instructions for use in the text field.

Enter *Infuse over 60 minutes.*

Note: These default instructions may be changed when filling the prescription, if needed.

18 Click on the **SAVE** 🖫 icon located at the top right of the toolbar. Basic information regarding the new compound has been saved to the *Drugs* form. You are now ready to add the ingredients of the new compound to the *Drugs* form. The bottom section of the *Drugs* form has three tabbed pages: (1) yellow tab—*Manufacturing & Available NDCs*; (2) green tab—*Compounded Drug Ingredients*; and (3) blue tab—*3rd Party NDC Preferences*.

Click the GREEN TAB to select COMPOUNDED DRUG INGREDIENTS.

19 The IV solution and the chemotherapy drug additive and amount needed will be added one at a time to the grid. Click on the **NEW** 🗋 icon located at the bottom right of this *Drugs* form. Two dialog boxes pop up on the screen: *Drug Name Lookup* and *Compound Drug Ingredients*.

20   Key in the first few letters of the desired diluents or IV solution being used. Select the correct drug from the list by clicking on the drug name. Click **OK**.

> **Enter *Sod* for sodium chloride 0.9% IV solution and the quantity of *500 ml* (base fluid).**

21   Click on the **SAVE** 🖫 icon on the bottom of the *Compound Drug Ingredients* dialog box.

22   Now add the chemotherapy drug or additive by clicking on the **NEW** 🗋 icon located at the bottom right of this *Drugs* form. Review steps 19 through 21 to add each ingredient.

> **Enter *Eto* for Etoposide 20 mg/ml, 5 ml vial.**
>
> **Calculate the amount of milliliters needed from the order provided.**
>
> **In this case, the quantity is 10 ml.**

23   Click the **CALCULATE** icon located at the bottom right of the window. Now you have completed the task of adding a new IV chemotherapy order to the pharmacy computer system! Click on the **CLOSE** 🗗 icon located at the top right of the toolbar.

24   Perform a drug look-up to make sure the new compound has been correctly added to the computer system.

25   Click on **DATA** from the toolbar located on the top of the screen.

26   Select **DRUGS** from the drop-down menu.

27   Click on the **FIND** 🔍 icon located at the top left of the toolbar.

28   The *Drug Name Lookup* dialog box appears.

> **Enter *ETO* to search for Etoposide 200 mg/NS 500 ml, or use the quick code you selected, *ETO200IV*.**

29   Select the correct compound from the list by clicking on the drug name. Click **OK**.

30   Read through the *Drugs* form to check for accuracy. Click on the **CLOSE** 🗗 icon on the top right of the toolbar to clear the screen.

31   Prepare and print the label based on the patient information on the medication order at the beginning of the lab.

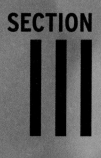

REPORTS

LAB
16

Control Drug Report

Steps to Create a Control Drug Report

1 Access the main screen of Visual SuperScript.

2 Click on **REPORTS** from the menu toolbar located at the top of the screen.

3 Select **DRUG REPORTS** from the drop-down menu. Then select **CONTROL DRUG REPORT** from the expanded menu.

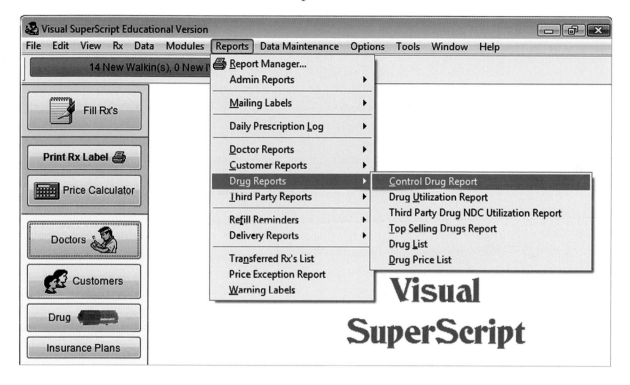

4 The *Control Drug Report* dialog box appears. Notice that the insertion point is in the first data entry field, **DATE FROM**. Key in the date that the *Control Drug Report* should start.

Key in *01/01/2005*.

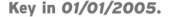

HINT: Deleting the default date that appears in the data entry field is not necessary. The date that is keyed in will replace the existing default date.

5   Key in the date that the *Control Drug Report* should end in the **To** data
    entry field.

Key in *03/01/2005*.

6   The **DRUG SELECTION** field will designate if the report will generate a
    list of Class/Schedule II drugs only: **C2 ONLY**; Class/Schedule III through
    Class/Schedule V: **C3-C5** drugs; or **ALL (C3-C5)** drugs. Click on the
    appropriate choice.

Select All (C2-C5).

7   The **SORT BY** field will designate the order in which the report should
    be arranged. Indicate how the report should be arranged: **FILL DATE**,
    DRUG NAME, or **CUSTOMER**. Click on the appropriate choice.

Select DRUG NAME.

8   Choose the appropriate **REPORT LAYOUT**.

Select DETAIL.

9   Click on **PREVIEW** located at the bottom of the *Control Drug Report*
    dialog box. The selected *Control Drug Report* will open and appear on the
    screen.

```
                              DAA EDUCATIONAL SOFTWARE              PAGE NO:  1
                      369 HARVARD ST, SUITE 1,BROOKLINE, MA 02446   DATE:07/05/11
                                    (617) 734-7366


                            Controlled Drugs Report For Sched 2-5
                                   (01/01/05  To 03/01/05)


    Rx#  OrigDate  FillDate  Ref    Customer         Doctor            Drug              Qty    RPh    DEA#

    386592 01/23/05 01/23/05 0/0  THOMAS, CHARLES    XAVIER, FRANCIS   ACETAMINOPHEN-COD #3   30.00 KAP   AX5565532
    Trip Serial#:
    386538 01/12/05 01/12/05 0/2  WINTERS, JOHN      ADAMS, JOHN       ALPRAZOLAM 0.5 MG TABLET  62.00 AB    AA5041710
    Trip Serial#:
    386538 01/12/05 02/12/05 1/2  WINTERS, JOHN      ADAMS, JOHN       ALPRAZOLAM 0.5 MG TABLET  62.00 AB    AA5041710
    Trip Serial#:
    386671 02/15/05 02/15/05 0/2  BANASKEY, ELZORA   SMITH, WILLIAM J. ALPRAZOLAM 0.5 MG TABLET  62.00 AB    AS2456324
    Trip Serial#:
    201817 08/31/04 01/10/05 2/3  ABSTON, KINLEY B   WATSON, JAMES     DIAZEPAM 10 MG TABLET     60.00 AB    AW6632182
    Trip Serial#:
    201817 08/31/04 01/31/05 2/3  ABSTON, KINLEY B   WATSON, JAMES     DIAZEPAM 10 MG TABLET     60.00 AB    AW6632182
    Trip Serial#:
    201817 08/31/04 01/10/05 1/3  ABSTON, KINLEY B   WATSON, JAMES     DIAZEPAM 10 MG TABLET     60.00 AB    AW6632182
    Trip Serial#:
    386562 01/18/05 01/18/05 0/0  OGG, DONALD        ALI, SYED RIAZ    DIAZEPAM 2 MG TABLET     100.00 KAP   AA3221140
    Trip Serial#:
    386623 02/04/05 02/04/05 0/0  POSNER, ROSE       IZBITSKY, JOSEPH  FLURAZEPAM 30 MG CAPSULE  30.00 KAP   AI1465665
    Trip Serial#:
    386527 01/09/05 01/09/05 0/0  MAY, CORNELIA D    DRAIME, ROBERT    FOCALIN 2.5 MG TABLET     60.00 AB    AD2993980
    Trip Serial#:1111111
    386660 02/11/05 02/11/05 0/0  TEDFORD, HAZEL     REAGAN, R.        FOCALIN 2.5 MG TABLET     60.00 AB    AR8843319
    Trip Serial#:1111111
    386651 02/09/05 02/09/05 0/0  DUKE, MICHAEL      HARDY, STEPHEN    GUAIFENESIN W/CODEINE    120.00 KAP   AH4442149
    Trip Serial#:
    386658 02/11/05 02/11/05 0/2  JORDAN, MICHELLE   DAVIS, KAREN      HYDROCODONE/APAP 10/325   30.00 AB    AD4252261
```

10   Click on the **PRINT REPORT** icon located at the top right of the *Report Designer* toolbar.

11   Click on the **CLOSE PREVIEW** icon located at the top right of the *Report Designer* toolbar. The report is closed out and the *Control Drug Report* dialog box returns.

Exercise

Scenario

The managing pharmacist is reconciling the CII logbook. A discrepancy is in methylphenidate, 5 mg. The CII logbook indicates that the pharmacy should have 140 tablets in stock. However, the physical count of methylphenidate 5 mg is 160 tablets. The managing pharmacist has asked for your help in finding out where the discrepancy between the CII logbook and the actual medication in stock occurred.

Task

Following the steps from the *Drug Reports: Control Drug Report* exercise, compile a detailed listing of dispensed methylphenidate 5 mg from 01/01/2005 to 03/01/2005. Print the report and submit it for verification.

1   What is the number of methylphenidate 5 mg tablets that were dispensed from the pharmacy between 01/08/2005 and 02/13/2005?

2   What are the three *Control Drug Report* sort choices?

Quick Challenge

You are becoming more familiar with the Visual SuperScript software system. Can you find the main menu option that will print a list of top-selling drugs?

1   Print a *Top-Selling Drug Report* listing the 10 top-selling drugs by average wholesale price (AWP) from 01/01/2005 through 06/30/2005. Submit the report for verification.

2   What is the name of the top-selling or top-performing drugs for this time period?

Daily Prescription Log Report

LAB OBJECTIVES

In this lab, you will:

- Learn how to create a report that summarizes the pharmacy dispensing records. Many states require a hard copy of all electronic records to be kept on file at the pharmacy.

STUDENT DIRECTIONS

Estimated completion time: 20 minutes

1. Read through the steps in the lab before performing the lab exercise.
2. After reading through the lab, perform the required steps to generate a daily prescription log report.
3. Complete the exercise at the end of the lab.

Steps to Create a Daily Prescription Log Report

1   Access the main screen of Visual SuperScript.

2   Click on **REPORTS** from the menu toolbar located at the top of the screen.

3   Select **DAILY PRESCRIPTION LOG** from the drop-down menu. Then select **DAILY RX LOG** from the expanded menu.

4   The *Daily Rx Log* dialog box appears. The **SELECT** section of the dialog box offers three choices on information that will be included in the *Daily Prescription Log Report*: **ALL PRESCRIPTIONS**, **NEW PRESCRIPTIONS ONLY**, or **REFILLS ONLY**. Click on the appropriate choice.

Select *All Prescriptions.*

5   Key in the desired date range in the **INCLUDE RECORDS FROM** field.

Key in *11/01/2005* to *12/31/2005.*

6   The **AGGREGATION TYPE** field allows for formatting choices in the report. Click on the appropriate choice.

> **HINT:** Choose **SEPARATE EACH DAY** if the report should have prescription information from each date on a separate page. Choose **COMBINED FOR PERIOD** if the report should have prescription information flow from one page to another, regardless of the date.

Choose *Separate Each Day.*

7   Choose the amount of information that should be included on the Daily Prescription Log report in the **DETAIL LEVEL** section of the *Daily Rx Log* dialog box. Click on the appropriate choice.

> **HINT:** **DETAIL LEVEL ONE** is the basic report providing prescription information. **DETAIL LEVEL TWO** provides the patient address in addition to the basic information. **DETAIL LEVEL THREE** provides patient and prescriber address, as well as the National Drug Code (NDC) number of the dispensed medication in addition to the basic information.

Choose *Detail Level Three.*

8 Click on the **Show Cost Using** check box. Designate if the report should be generated to show the average wholesale price (**AWP**) for prescriptions dispensed during the selected date(s) or the **Acquisition** cost of the medications dispensed. Click on the appropriate choice.

Select *AWP.*

9 The **Sort by Section** of the dialog box allows four different formats in sorting or arranging the *Daily Prescription Log* report: **Fill Date**, **Drug Class**, **Rx #**, or **Pay type**. Click on the appropriate choice.

Choose *Fill Date.*

10 Click on **Preview** located on the bottom of the *Daily Rx Log* dialog box. The selected *Daily Prescription Log Report* will open and appear on the screen.

```
                          DAA EDUCATIONAL SOFTWARE                    PAGE NO:  1
                369 HARVARD ST, SUITE 1,BROOKLINE, MA 02446
                               (617) 734-7366                         DATE:07/05/11



               Rx LOG SORTED BY DISPENSE DATE:(11/01/05 To 12/31/05)


  _____
  Customer              Doctor Name/        Drug/NDC/Drugclass/       Fill
  Name/Address          Dea#/Address        Prescribed Drug   Rx#     Date   Ref  RPh   Qty   Price  Copay  InsPlan
  ABSTON, KINLEY B  JONES, STANLEY(AS2334453) LANOXICAPS 0.05 MG CAPSUL 386913 11/09/05  0/0  AB   60.0   27.19  27.19
  201 MAPLE ST          23 CENTER STREET    00173-0270-55   (RX)
  CAMBRIDGE,MA          CHESTNUT HILL,MA 02167  LANOXICAPS 0.05 MG CAPSUL
  _____
                                    Total  Copay:       27.19
  _____

       _____      _____     _____
      | NEW:       1       |    | REFILL:      0     |   | TOTAL:       1      |
  NEW:| INCOME:    27.19   |REFILLS:| INCOME:   0.00 |TOTAL:| INCOME:   27.19  |
      | MARGIN:    11.02   |    | MARGIN:    0.00    |   | MARGIN:    11.02    |
       _____      _____     _____


            The above listed prescriptions were dispensed on the date shown.


         _____          _____
         Pharmacist                           Date
```

11   Click on the **PRINT REPORT** icon located at the top right of the *Report Designer* toolbar. Be sure to print only the pages necessary for this report.

12   Click on the **CLOSE REPORT** icon located at the top right of the *Report Designer* toolbar. The report is closed out and the *Daily Rx Log* dialog box returns.

13   Click on the **CLOSE** ⏻ icon located at the bottom of the *Daily Rx Log* dialog box.

Exercise

Scenario

The pharmacy manager has asked you to compile a report that summarizes the prescriptions dispensed the previous month (May 2005). The manager would like the report arranged by third-party payers. The report should include the NDC number of the dispensed drug. The manager has also told you that the report will be filed as a hard-copy record or backup record in case of system failure.

Task

Following the steps presented in this lab, compile a *Daily Prescription Log Report* that will meet the pharmacy manager's needs. Print the report and submit it for verification.

1 Who are the third-party payers in May 2005?

2 What was the fill date for the One-Touch Test Strips?

3 Are the One-Touch Test Strips listed as OTC or Rx?

Quick Challenge

1 You are now familiar with the steps of generating a business report. Can you compile a *Profit Summary Report* for October 2005? Submit the printed report for verification.

HINT: Select an item by left-clicking on the item with your mouse.

LAB
18

Customer History Report

In this lab, you will:

- Learn how to create a pharmacy business report that details the patient/customer prescription history.

Estimated completion time: 15 minutes

1. Read through the steps in the lab before performing the lab exercise.
2. After reading through the lab, perform the required steps to generate a customer history report.
3. Complete the exercise at the end of the lab.

Steps to Create a Customer History Report

1 Access the main screen of Visual SuperScript.

2 Click on **REPORTS** from the menu toolbar located at the top of the screen.

3 Select **CUSTOMER REPORTS** from the drop-down menu. Then select **CUSTOMER HISTORY** from the expanded menu.

4 The *Customer History* dialog box appears. Notice that the insertion point is in the first data entry field, **DATE FROM**. Key in the date that the *Customer History Report* should start. Deleting the default date that appears in the data entry field is not necessary. The date that is keyed in will replace the existing default date.

Key in *01/20/2005.*

5 Key in the date that the *Customer History Report* should end in the **To** data entry field.

Key in *12/31/2005.*

6 The **SHOW** field will designate whether the report should be generated to show the **COPAY** amount for the medications or the actual **PRICE** of the medications. Click on the appropriate choice.

Select *Copay.*

7 The **FORMAT** field will designate whether the report should be generated in an **INSURANCE** format or a **NHOME** (nursing home) format. Select **INSURANCE** format unless the patient is a resident of a nursing home. Click on the appropriate choice.

Select *Insurance.*

8 Select the **NEW PAGE FOR EACH CUSTOMER** field if individual pages are desired.

9 The **FOR** data field offers several different choices in generating the *Customer History Report*. Select one of the five choices in which the *Customer History Report* will be generated. Click on the appropriate choice.

Select *Individual Customer.*

10 The **NAME** data entry field will ask for the customer name or the name of the insurance plan. The required information depends on the selection made in step 9. Key in the appropriate information.

Key in *Posner, Rose.*

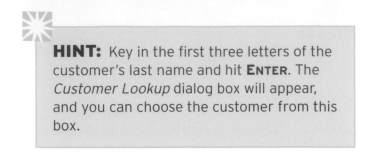

HINT: Key in the first three letters of the customer's last name and hit **ENTER**. The *Customer Lookup* dialog box will appear, and you can choose the customer from this box.

11   Choose the print layout for the report.

Select *Portrait*.

12   Click on **PREVIEW** located the bottom of the *Customer History* dialog
box. The selected Customer History Report will open and appear on the
screen.

DAA EDUCATIONAL SOFTWARE
369 HARVARD ST, SUITE 1, BROOKLINE, MA 02446
(617) 734-7366

PAGE NO: 1
DATE:07/05/11

Customer History Report For POSNER, ROSE
(01/20/05 To 12/31/05)

Rx#	FillDate	Ref#	Doctor	Drug	NDC#	Qty	Copay	InsPlan	Auth #
386623	02/04/05	0	ISBITSKY, JOSEPH	FLURASEPAM 30 MG	00143-3370-01	30.00	5.00		
386624	02/04/05	0	ISBITSKY, JOSEPH	CELEBREX 100 MG	00025-1520-31	50.00	10.00		

TOTAL $15.00

WE APPRECIATE YOUR BUSINESS.

SIGNED: R.Ph.

---

13   Click on the **PRINT REPORT** icon located at the top right of the *Report
Designer* toolbar.

14   Click on the **CLOSE PREVIEW** icon located at the top right of the *Report
Designer* toolbar. The report is closed out and the *Customer History* dialog
box returns.

Exercise

Scenario

It is January 10, 2006. Mr. Harry Zinn calls your pharmacy asking
for a detailed listing of the medications that he purchased during
the previous year. Harry Zinn explains that he needs the detailed
medication record to complete his income tax report for 2005.

Task

Following the steps from the *Reporting Customer History* exercise, compile a detailed listing of Mr. Harry Zinn's medications for the year 2005. Print the report and submit it for verification.

1   What was the total out-of-pocket expense that Mr. Zinn paid to your pharmacy in 2005 for prescription medications?

2   How many tablets did Mr. Zinn receive on his 04/06/2005 prescription for Celebrex?

ASSESSMENT

LAB
19

Community Pharmacy Comprehensive Exercise

LAB OBJECTIVES

In this lab, you will:

- Use the skills learned to perform necessary computer functions to enter a new prescription into a pharmacy system and process it for customer pickup.
- Use the skills learned to process refills and process them for customer pickup.
- Use the knowledge gained to simulate real tasks such as prior approvals, refill authorization, billing, and verification of correct patient and medications that are performed in a community setting.

STUDENT DIRECTIONS

Estimated completion time: 120 minutes

1. Use the prescriptions provided in this lab to simulate the processes of preparing medications for customers.
2. Interpret the new prescriptions, input the data, and prepare labels, as well as perform adjudication for insurance and process cash transactions.
3. Refills should be processed from the list of calls received from the patients.
4. Once completed, assemble the stock bottle, the prepared medication, the original prescription (if applicable), and any other documentation required for your instructor to check.

> **HINT:** Use verifying information, such as the patient's birth date or address, to identify the correct patient when searching. You may refer to the Community lab section.

New Prescriptions

R̶x

Dr. John Smith
739 Stockton Street
Waltham, MA 02454
Office: (781) 333-2121
Fax: (617) 734-6340

Patient Name: _____ Holly Bean _____

Date: _____ 2/17/2012 _____

Address: ___ 96 Milk Street, Newton, MA 02456 _____

Refill: ___ 0 ____
Rx: ___ amoxil 875 mg #30 1 tab pot id x 3 days ___

DEA: AS3456325
State License: 2724141

R̶x

Dr. Jasmine Abbosh
836 Farmington Avenue
Worcester, MA 01601
Office: (617) 232-9911
Fax: (617) 734-6340

Patient Name: _____ Richard Clemens _____

Date: _____ 2/17/2012 _____

Address: ___ 345 Fenwick Dr, Chestnut Hill, MA 02167 _____

Refill: ___ 0 ____
Rx: ___ Zpak #1 2 tabs po now, then 1 tab po qd x 4 days ___
        Brand necessary

DEA: BA4884533

℞

Dr. Kareem Babu
300 Stainford Street
Springfield, MA 01104
Office: (413) 776-9000
Fax: (413) 776-9001

Patient Name: _____ Larry Jones _____

Date: _____ 2/17/2012 _____

Address: _____ 63 Birch Street, Wellesley, MA 02482 _____

       Refill: ___ 0 ___
       Rx: ___ Bactroban 2% ung 22 g tube AAA bid ud ___

DEA: BB5723469
State License: 2724141

℞

Dr. Antoine Diallo
5500 Maryland Street
Bethesda, MA 20814
Office: (301) 725-3458
Fax: (301) 725-3458

Patient Name: _____ Miguel Sanchez _____

Date: _____ 2/17/2012 _____

Address: _____ 75 Tremont Street, Cambridge, MA 02139 _____

       Refill: ___ 3 ___
       Rx: ___ Humulin R inject 15 units sq tid ac ___
           (Spanish label required)

DEA: AD1234567

℞

Dr. Stephen Hardy
76 Walnut Street
Allston, MA 02134
Office: (617) 532-6390
Fax: (617) 734-6340

Patient Name: _____ Margaret Noonan

Date: _____ 2/17/2012

Address: _____ 30 Inman Street, Brighton, MA 02135

Refill: ___ 0

Rx: _____ etanercept 25 mg kit #1 ud

DEA: AH4442149RES
State License: 4525253

℞

Dr. Robert Cornish
1789 Hyde Avenue
Allston, MA 02134
Office: (617) 372-7650
Fax: (617) 734-6340

Patient Name: _____ Bernice Good

Date: _____ 2/17/2012

Address: _____ 92 Fernwood Terrace, Allston, MA 02134

Refill: ___ 0 ud

Rx: _____ Blood glucose meter, lancets, strips

DEA: ACS5433230
State License: 7665899

℞

Dr. Karen Davis
132 Hines Street
Newton, MA 02456
Office: (617) 553-4300
Fax: (617) 734-6340

Patient Name: _____ Verna Bushey _____

Date: _____ 2/17/2012 _____

Address: __ 68 Birch Street, Newton, MA 02456 _____

      Refill: ___ 0 ___
      Rx: ___ Compazine 25 mg supp #XII 1 pr bid for n/v ___

DEA: AD4252261
State License: 3562215

℞

Dr. Dennis Feldman
306 E. 76th Street
New York, NY 10011
Refills: (212) 665-5433
Fax: (212) 665-5433

Patient Name: _____ Lloyd Bean _____

Date: _____ 2/17/2012 _____

Address: __ 96 Milk Street, Newton, MA 02456 _____

      Refill: ___ 2 ___
      Rx: ___ Tagamet 300 mg/5 ml disp 480 ml sig: 800 mg hs ___

DEA: BF5178562
State License: 93599127

Refills Requested

If refill numbers are not provided or if you are unclear about what a patient has requested, then verify all requests with your instructor before filling. In some cases, the medication name or simply the classification has been given.

1. **Bruce Babbage**
   DOB: 6/17/35
   Refill requested: 201114, eye drops, and 201585

2. **Patricia Armstrong**
   DOB: 8/14/87
   Refill requested: GERD medication

3. **Francis Preston**
   DOB: 5/23/46
   Refill requested: 388101, 388102

4. **Ronald Gaston**
   Address: Laker Street
   Refill requested: Viagra, nasal spray, and 386873

5. **Frank Bosworth**
   DOB: 3/15/11
   Refill requested: folic acid, 201575, and 201576

6. **Michelle Jordan**
   Address: Elm Street
   Refill requested: 386728

7. **James Rowen**
   DOB: 6/3/62
   Refill requested: muscle relaxer and steroid pack

Institutional Pharmacy Comprehensive Exercise

LAB OBJECTIVES

In this lab, you will:

- Use the skills learned to perform necessary computer functions to enter new intravenous orders into a pharmacy system.
- Use the knowledge gained to simulate real tasks, such as interpreting orders, using references for dilutions and storage, and using proper mixing techniques, performed in a hospital or institutional setting.

STUDENT DIRECTIONS

Use the following orders to simulate the processes of compounding sterile medications for hospital patients. You will interpret the physician's orders, input the data, and prepare labels for the intravenous medications ONLY. Use any approved reference to determine additional information needed. Once completed, your instructor may also ask you to prepare the intravenous medications using the aseptic technique previously learned in your program.

HINT: Use verifying information, such as birthdate or room number, to identify the correct patient when searching the database. You may refer to Section II: Institutional Pharmacy Practice for additional help.

Patient name	Ellis, Floyd		Diet	Weight	Height
Room number	Med Surg #1		as tol	202	5'7
Hospital number	24221		Diagnosis		
Attending Physician	Dr. Takanori Ozawa		COPD, Pneumonia, diabetes		
			Drug Allergies PCN		

DATE	TIME		
11/24/11	1115 AM	Admit to Med-Surg (Dr.	
		Condition: guarded	
		Vitals: as per protocol	
		Activity: As tolerated	
		Nursing: FSBG QAC, QHS sliding scale	
		O² via NC to maintain sat ≥ 92%	
		Labs: CBC, chem 22	
		Chest x-ray PA, lateral	
		CBC in AM	
		Meds: Rocephin 1g IV qday (1st dose 11-22-11)	
		Solu medrol 80mg IV q6h	
		Azithromycin 500mg IV qday	
		Albuterol nebs 1 dose q6hrs	
		Atrovent nebs 1 dose q6hrs	
		Albuterol nebs 1 dose q2hrs prn wheezing	
		or dyspnea	
		Singulair 10mg po qday	
		Glucophage 500mg po bid	
		Glipizide 5mg po bid	
		Neurontin 400mg po tid	
		Requip 0.5mg po BID	
		Zantac 150mg po bid	
		Dr. Ozawa	

Patient name	Anna Saba		Diet	Weight	Height
Room number	114		1800 cal	142	5'3
Hospital number	32112		Diagnosis		
Attending Physician	Dr. R. Zimmerman		OB, R/o Ovarian cysts		
			Drug Allergies NKA		

DATE	TIME		
1/28/11	1420	Discontinue Phenergan (hx of making	
		patient confused)	
		Zofran 4 mg IV q4 hrs prn N÷V	
		v/o Dr. Zimmerman K Davis, RN 1330	
		1/28/11	

Patient name	Ben Tulley	7-1-01	Diet	Weight	Height
Room number 420			Reg	101	4'9
Hospital number 13429			Diagnosis		
Attending Physician Robert Clear, MD.			MRSA?		
			Drug Allergies Sulfa		

DATE	TIME		
11/27/11	1128	Give dose of Rocephin 1g IVPB now.	
		√o Dr. Clear. KDas, RN 1104 11/27/11	

Patient name Hazel Tedford. 8-30-23			Diet	Weight	Height
Room number 115			Low NA	89	4'7
Hospital number 34211			Diagnosis		
Attending Physician Dr. J. Goffrey			Lower Resp Tract infection, R/o septicemia		
			Drug Allergies NKDA		
DATE	TIME				
11/26	0550	1g Rocephin IV now, then q24h			
		D/C Levaquin			
		PA and lateral of chest			
		up right Abd. X-ray			
		RBTO Dr. Goffrey / K Davis, RN.			
		11/26/11 @ 0555			

Patient name	Samuel Urban 9-2-58		Diet		Weight	Height
Room number 301			GS tol		172	6'1
Hospital number 32113			Diagnosis			
Attending Physician Dr J. Rose			Plop pain, unknown origin			
			Drug Allergies NKA			

DATE	TIME		
11-30-11	1330	① Nubain 10 mg IM X 1 now	
		Dr. Rose	

Sig Abbreviation Shortcuts

ABBREVIATION	MEANING
1-2	1 or 2
1-2G	1 or 2 drops
1 APP	1 applicator
1C	1 capsule
1CBID	Take 1 capsule twice each day
1CQD	Take 1 capsule daily
1CQID	Take 1 capsule four times a day
1CTID	Take 1 capsule three times a day
1DR	Take 1 teaspoon
1G	1 drop
1IAPP	Insert 1 applicator
1SSTS	Take $1\frac{1}{2}$ teaspoon
1T	1 tablet
1TBID	1 tablet twice a day
1TPOBID	1 tablet by mouth twice a day
1TPOQD	1 tablet by mouth each day
1TPOQDHS	1 tablet by mouth every day at bedtime
1TQD	1 tablet each day
1TQID	1 tablet four times a day
1TTID	1 tablet three times a day
2C	2 capsules
2G	2 drops
2T	2 tablets
3G	3 drops
3TSP	3 teaspoons
4G	4 drops
4HRS	4 hours
AA	Affected area; Amino acid solution
AAA	Apply to affected area
AAD	After dinner
AAS	After supper
AC	Before meals
AE	Into the affected eye
AM	Morning
AND	And

ABBREVIATION	MEANING
AP	Apply
ASAP	As soon as possible
ATC	Around the clock
BID	Twice a day
BM	Bowel movement
BOLUS	Intravenous push
BP	Blood pressure
BRP	Bathroom priv.
C	With
CAP	Capsule
CCM	With food or milk
CF	With food
CM	With meals
D_5W	Dextrose 5% in water
D_5 1/4 N.S.	Dextrose 5% in 1/4 normal saline
D_5 0.2% NACL	Dextrose 5% in 0.2% sodium chloride
D_5 1/2 N.S.	Dextrose 5% in 1/2 normal saline
D_5 0.45% NACL	Dextrose 5% in 0.45% sodium chloride
D_5 N.S.	Dextrose 5% in normal saline
D_5 0.9% NACL	Dextrose 5% in 0.9% sodium chloride
D_5LR	Dextrose 5% in lactated Ringer's solution
$D_{10}W$	Dextrose 10% in water
$D_{20}W$	Dextrose 20% in water
$D_{30}W$	Dextrose 30% in water
$D_{40}W$	Dextrose 40% in water
$D_{50}W$	Dextrose 50% in water
$D_{70}W$	Dextrose 70% in water
D	Daily
D1T	Dissolve 1 tablet
DA	Dissolve and
DAY	Day
DIA	Diarrhea
DIS	Dissolve
DISP	Dispense
DR	Drink
DX	Diagnosis
DWW	Dilute with water
EN	Each nostril
EVERY	Every
F	For
F1	For 1 week
F10	For 10 days
F14	For 14 days
F2	For 2 weeks
F5	For 5 days
F7	For 7 days
FE	For external use only
FIN	Finished
FP	For pain
FX	Fracture

ABBREVIATION	MEANING
GTT	Drop
GTTS	Drops
(H)	Hypodermic
H, HR	Hour
HA	Headache
HOUR	Hour
I	Instill
I1G	Instill 1 drop
I1P	Inhale 1 puff
I1S	Insert 1 suppository
I1T	Insert 1 tablet
I2G	Instill 2 drops
I2P	Inhale 2 puffs
I3G	Instill 3 drops
I3P	Inhale 3 puffs
I4G	Instill 4 drops
I4P	Inhale 4 puffs
I5G	Instill 5 drops
ID	Intradermal
IM	Intramuscular
INFECT	Infection
IL	In liquids
INF	For infection
INS	Insert
IT	Intrathecal
ITCH	Itching
IV	Intravenous
IVP	Intravenous push
IVPB	IV piggyback
IVSS	IV soluset
IW	In water
L	Left
LE	Left ear
LR (RL)	Lactated Ringer's solution (Ringer's lactated solution)
MR	May repeat
N	Nerves
NF	Nonformulary
NKA	No known allergies
NPO	Nothing by mouth
NR	No refill
N.S.	Normal saline
NV	Nausea and vomiting
(O)	Orally
OA	Into affected eye
P	For pain, after
PIT	Place 1 tablet
PA	Pain
PAC	Packet
PATCH	Patch

ABBREVIATION	MEANING
PC	After meals
PL	Place
PM	Afternoon
PO	By mouth
PR	Rectally
PRN	As needed
PRNA	As needed for anxiety
PRNC	As needed for cough
PRND	As needed for diarrhea
PRNF	As needed for
PRNHA	As needed for headache
PRNP	As needed for pain
PV	Vaginally
Q	Every
Q12H	Every 12 hours
Q3-4H	Every 3 to 4 hours
Q4-6H	Every 4 to 6 hours
Q4H	Every 4 hours
Q6-8H	Every 6 to 8 hours
Q6H	Every 6 hours
Q8H	Every 8 hours
QAM	Every morning
QH	Every hour
QID	Four times a day
QNOC	Every night
QOH	Every other hour
QPM	Every evening
QS	Sufficient quantity
QSAD	Sufficient quantity to add
R	Right
RE	Right ear
RX	Take, recipe
S	Suppository, without
S2D	Squirt twice daily
SIG	Label
SL	Under tongue
SSAP	$\frac{1}{2}$ applicator
SSTSP	$\frac{1}{2}$ teaspoon
STAT	Immediately
SUB-Q	Subcutaneously
SX	Surgery
T	Take
T1	Take 1
T1C	Take 1 capsule
T1-2C	Take 1 or 2 capsules
T1-2T	Take 1 or 2 tablets
T1SST	Take 1$\frac{1}{2}$ tablets
TID	Three times a day
T1TBL	Take 1 tablespoonful
T1TBS	Take 1 tablespoonful

ABBREVIATION	MEANING
T1TSP	Take 1 teaspoonful
T2	Take 2
T2C	Take 2 capsules
T2TSP	Take 2 teaspoons
T2T	Take 2 tablets
T3	Take 3
T3C	Take 3 capsules
T3T	Take 3 tablets
T3TSP	Take 3 teaspoons
T4C	Take 4 capsules
T4T	Take 4 tablets
T4TSP	Take 4 teaspoons
T5C	Take 5 capsules
T5T	Take 5 tablets
TAKE	Take
TBID	Take 1 tablet twice a day
TBL	Tablespoonful
TBSP	Tablespoonful
THEN	Then
TID	Three times a day
TK	Take
TLA	To large area
TOP	Topically
TPN	Total parenteral nutrition
TRA	To run at
TSP	Teaspoonful
TSST	Take $1/2$ tablet
TUD	Take as directed
TTSP	Take $1/2$ teaspoonful
U2I	Use 2 inhalations
U2P	Use 2 puffs
U2S	Use 2 sprays
UAT	Until all taken
UD	As directed, unit dose
UF	Until finished
UG	Until gone
USE	Use
USP	United States Pharmacopeia
UUD	Use as directed
VAG	Vaginally
W/A	While awake
WF	With food
WJ	With juice
WM	With meals
WMB	With meals and bedtime
WW	With water

Community Prescriptions

Exercise

Process the following prescriptions. Once each prescription is processed, print the medication label, pull the medication from stock, and prepare the medication bottle.

Dr. Jasmine Abbosh
836 Farmington Avenue
Worcester, MA.01601
860-232-9911
BA4892433

For: Floyd Ellis

Address: 73 Birch St. Worcester, MA.   Date: 3/21/11

Glucophage 500 mg ÷ qd #30
Folic Acid ÷ mg #30
Inderal 40 mg ÷ bid #60
Zyloprim 300 mg ÷ qd #30

REFILL __4__ TIMES   Dr. Jasmine Abbosh

                                                    M.D.

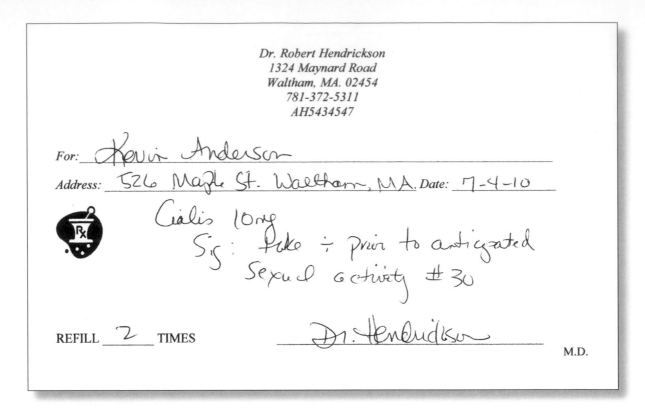

Dr. Robert Hendrickson
1324 Maynard Road
Waltham, MA. 02454
781-372-5311
AH5434547

For: Kevin Anderson

Address: 526 Maple St. Waltham, MA. *Date:* 7-4-10

Cialis 10mg
Sig: take ½ prior to anticipated
sexual activity #30

REFILL __2__ TIMES   Dr. Hendrickson

M.D.

Dr. Jasmine Abbosh
836 Farmington Avenue
Worcester, MA.01601
860-232-9911
BA4892433

For: Maxine Broswell

Address: 75 Pinewood Terr Worcester   *Date:* 6-6-10

Humira 40mg
Sig: inj subcutaneous q every other week

REFILL __0__ TIMES   Dr. Jasmine Abbosh

M.D.

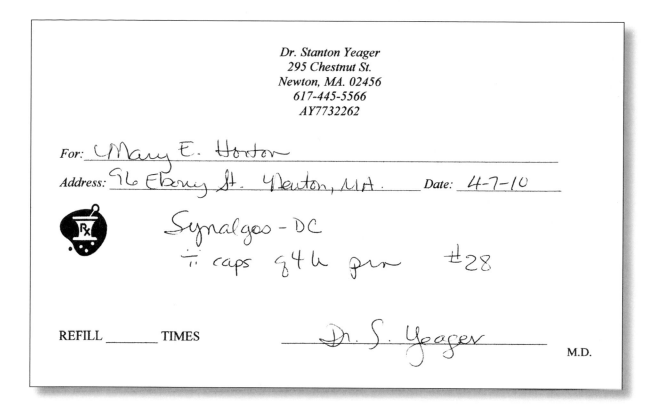

Dr. Stanton Yeager
295 Chestnut St.
Newton, MA. 02456
617-445-5566
AY7732262

For: Mary E. Horton

Address: 96 Ebony St. Newton, MA.   Date: 4-7-10

℞   Synalgos - DC
    ĩ caps q4h prn   #28

REFILL _____ TIMES   Dr. S. Yeager

M.D.

Dr. Earl Warren
123 Longwood Avenue
Wellesley, MA. 02482
781-237-4450
AW2222228

For: Jill Bottoms

Address: 21 Surrey St. West Roxbury   Date: 4-4-10

℞   Tamiflu susp 12mg/ml
    Disp. 45mg bid   pt. wt = 18 kg.

REFILL 0 TIMES   Dr. E. Warren

M.D.

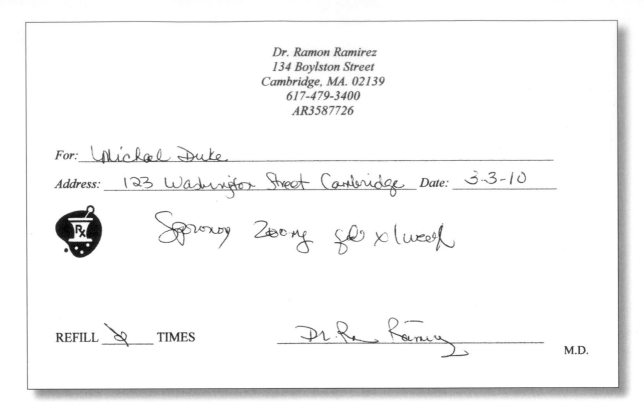

Dr. Ramon Ramirez
134 Boylston Street
Cambridge, MA. 02139
617-479-3400
AR3587726

For: _Michael Duke_

Address: _123 Washington Street Cambridge_ Date: _3-3-10_

℞ Spironoy 200mg gb x 1 week

REFILL _2_ TIMES   _Dr. Ra Ramirez_
                                                    M.D.

Dr. Terry Alexander
1756 Route 9D
Cold Springs, NY. 10516
845-265-1006
MA1407166

For: _Ernest Hatcher_

Address: _71 Poplar Street Cold Springs, NY_ Date: _6-6-10_

℞ Oxycontin 5mg q6h prn pain #24

"notify nursing home when ready"

REFILL _2_ TIMES   _Dr. Terry Alexander_
                                                    M.D.

Dr. Robert Hendrickson
1324 Maynard Road
Waltham, MA. 02454
781-372-5311
AH5434547

For: _Coryn Nardone_

Address: _381 Freeman St. Waltham, MA._   Date: _9-1-11_

℞   Cephalexin   500mg

Disp: #18

Sig: 2 Stat, then ÷ tid starting tomorrow

REFILL _x|_   TIMES   _Dr. Robert Hendrick._

M.D.

Dr. Ramon Ramirez
134 Boylston Street
Cambridge, MA. 02139
617-479-3400
AR3587726

For: _Patricia Armstrong_

Address: _23 Egmont St Cambridge, MA_   Date: _11-22-10_

℞   Prozac 20mg #60

Σ: ÷ AM, ÷ NOON pc

DESYREL 50mg   #30

Σ: ii or iii hs pc

REFILL _0_   TIMES   _Dr. Ram_

M.D.

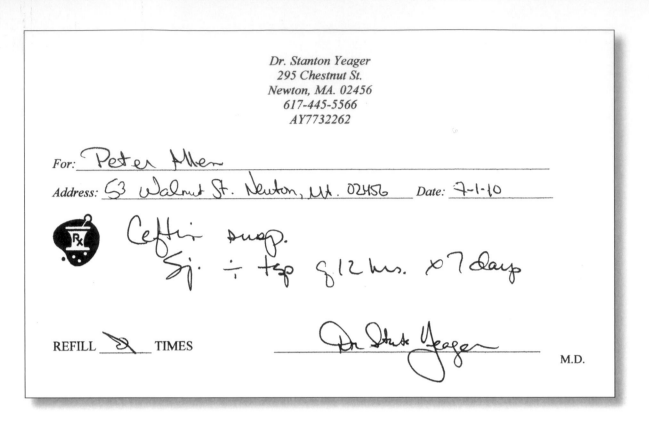

Nonsterile Extemporaneous Compound Prescriptions

Exercise

Process the following prescriptions. Once each prescription is processed, print the medication label, pull the medication from stock, and prepare the medication bottle.

Dr. John Burns
123 Main Street
Brighton, MA. 02135
617-456-7765
AB3623457

For: Samuel Urban

Address: 29 Walnut St. Brighton, MA.   Date: 8/22/10

GI Cocktail   60 mls
Mylanta, Lidocaine, Benadryl
Take As dir

REFILL __2__ TIMES   _____

M.D.

Dr. Ronald Zimmerman
609 Spruce Street
Chestnut Hill, MA.02167
617-445-5566
AZ2532118

For: Samuel Urban

Address: 29 Walnut St. Chestnut Hill, MA   Date: 12/12/10

RA Gel 100g

Ketoprofen 4% -4g
Gabapentin 5g
Baclofen 4g

REFILL _____ TIMES   Dr. R Zimmer

                                                        M.D.

Dr. Stanton Yeager
295 Chestnut St.
Newton, MA. 02456
617-445-5566
AY7732262

For: Carole Powers

Address: 3412 W. Lafayette Newton, MA.   Date: 12/17/10

ASA 3.6 g

Codeine sulfate 0.4 g
Mix and make #12 capsules

REFILL _____ TIMES   Dr. S. Yeager

                                                        M.D.

Dr. Alan Lamb
143 Babcock Street
Allston, MA.02134
617-212-5252
AL1234563

For: Sharon Peterson

Address: 70 Marlboro St. Allston, MA.   *Date:* 9/22/10

℞ MTMX Susp.

    100cc Mycostatin susp.   ii tsp po qid
    100cc Mylanta
    100cc Xylocaine (viscous)   #300ml
    Swish & Swallow

REFILL ___1___ TIMES

                                   M.D.

Dr. Stanton Yeager
295 Chestnut St.
Newton, MA. 02456
617-445-5566
AY7732262

For: Sarah King

Address: 246 Tamarac St. Newton, MA. *Date:* 2/19/11

℞ Dukes 120 ml

    Tetracycline 350 mg #3 caps
    Benadryl 12.5/5   #90 ml
    Nystatin Sup 100,000/ml   30 ml
    Hydrocortisone 2.5% cr   0.25 g

REFILL ___1___ TIMES   Dr. S. Yeager

                                   M.D.

Dr. Stanton Yeager
295 Chestnut St.
Newton, MA. 02456
617-445-5566
AY7732262

For: Todd Eusier

Address: 455 Ashburton Ln. Newton, MA *Date:* 2/2/11

Paragoric 30ml
Kaopectate q.s. ad 120ml
Mix well.

REFILL ___0___ TIMES   Dr. S. Yeager

M.D.

Intravenous Orders

Exercise

Process the following intravenous orders. Once each order is processed, print the medication label, pull the medication from stock, and prepare the medication.

Patient Name Ernest Hatcher	Diet Cl liq	Weight 180	Height 5'7"	BD: 3-27-29
Room Number 221-C	Diagnosis			
Hospital Number 47411 - Coolidge N.H.	Diverticulitis			
Attending Physician Dr. Terry Alexander	Drug Allergies NKA			

DATE	TIME		
3/5/10	0715	NS 1 ℓ @ 75 ml/hr Zosyn 3.375 g IVPB q 6 hr }	1st dose now
		Flagyl 500mg IVPB q 12 hrs }	1st dose now
		CBC, BMP in AM V/S q 4 hrs. Tylenol g ÷ po q 4 hr PRN T ≥ 101	
		Dr. Terry Alexander, MD. -0710	

Patient Name		Diet	Weight	Height	
Thelma Richey		Reg	129 lbs.	4"11	BD: 5-17-21
Room Number		Diagnosis			
321-B					
Hospital Number		Sepsis, R/o meningitis			
Coolidge Nursing Home					
Attending Physician		Drug Allergies			
Dr. Mark Owens		PCN, Sulfa			

DATE	TIME		
1/24/11	0730	Gentamycin 55mg / NS 50 ml IVPB now	
		Percocet 5mg po q6h prn pain	
		V/o KDavis RN.	
	1010	Admit to floor	
		Zantac 50mg / NS 50 ml x1 Bag	
		Bicitra 15 ml po x1	
		Reglan 10 mg IVP now	
		CXR in AM - portable	
		BMP, CBC, peak & trough in AM	
		I/0 q shift	
		Bedrest	
		V/o KDav RN	

Patient Name			Diet	Weight	Height
Mark Ianella 9-11-63			Reg as tol	129	60 in.
Room Number 422-B			Diagnosis		
Hospital Number 74113			Failure to thrive, dehydration		
Attending Physician Dr. Babu			Drug Allergies NKA		

DATE	TIME		

7/4/10	2200	Admit for observation
		Condition: guarded.
		Ensure apm admit.
		NS 1 ℓ @ 125 ml hr c̄ MVI
		Kdur ÷ po now
		CMP, CBC in Am
		chest CT SCAN now
		
		Levaquin 500 mg IVPB now and
		in Am
		vital signs q shift
		
		Demerol 25 mg q6 prn pain
		Phenergan 12.5 mg q6 prn nausea
		
		       V/o Dr. Babu
		        K Den, RN	

Patient Name Mary Harrison	Diet Reg	Weight 171 lb.	Height 5'5	BD: 6/13/20
Room Number CCU - 233	Diagnosis			
Hospital Number 45456	Pneumonia			
Attending Physician Dr. Larry Alexander	Drug Allergies NKA			

DATE	TIME		
3/3/10	1730	Admit to Floor	
		vitals q shift	
		Rocephin 500 mg / NS 50ml IV now	
		Xopenex neb q shift	
		Motrin 1 tsp. po tid	
		D5 1/4 NS c MVI @ 60ml/hr	
		CBC in Am	
		Dr. L. Alex	

Patient Name Gary Henderson		Diet 1600/no salt	Weight 490	Height 60 in.	BD: 4-30-47
Room Number 228-A		**Diagnosis**			
Hospital Number 53718		CHF, obesity, DM type II, asthma by hx			
Attending Physician Dr. Fenstermaker		**Drug Allergies** PCN			

DATE	TIME		
8/9/10	1750	admit to inpatient status	
		1) CBC, CMP, UA, thyroid panel lipid profile, BNP on admit	
		2) EKG	
		3) Xopenex 0.83mg qid	
		4) Lasix 40mg IV on admission	
		Meds:	
		Colace 100mg ÷ cap BID prn constipation	
		Glucovance 5mg ÷ BID po	
		Lipitor 20mg ÷ tab qhs po	
		Flovent 110mcg ÷ puffs bid	
		Norvasc 5mg ÷ tab po qd	
		Coreg 25mg ÷ tab po BID	
		Dr. Walter Fenstermaker, MD. -1756	

Chemotherapy Orders

Exercise

Process the following chemotherapy orders. Once each order is processed, print the medication label, pull the medication from stock, and prepare the medication.

CHEMOTHERAPY ORDERS

Date of order 4-7-10	Time of order 1400	Day 1 of this order 4-7	Patient diagnosis Ovarian CA
Pt name Allen, Mattie	Birth date 12-20-31	Cycle #	☒ Central Line ☐ Peripheral Line
Actual Weight 46 kg	Ideal Weight 50 kg	Adjusted Weight 41.7 kg	Height 145 cm	Body Surface Area 1.45 m²

CHEMOTHERAPY ORDERS: For each drug ordered below, fill in all boxes on the corresponding line or indicate n/a if not applicable.

Chemotherapy Drug	Rec dose	BSA/kg	Dose to be given	ROUTE	RATE	FREQUENCY or day #	# OF DOSES
Paraplatin	AUC=6		450 mg	IV	over 30 min	Day #1	1

PARAMETER(S)	Instructions (Check all that apply)	
	Call Case Mgr/Provider	HOLD
For absolute neutrophils count less than:	[ ]	[ ]
For platelets less than 100,000	[✓] RN Ellis, Mary	[ ]
For Mucositis Grade 3 or 4	[ ]	[ ]
For serum creatinine greater than:	[ ]	[ ]
Other:	[ ]	[ ]
Other:	[ ]	[ ]

Prescriber Signature (MD/PA-C/ARNP) Dr. Ronald Zimmerman	Attending MD Signature (*required prior to order submission*)
2nd Attending MD Signature (*required for non standard dose if documentation not available*)	Pharmacist Review Signature
Two RNs must verify dose of chemotherapy prior to administration of initial dose	Two RPhs must verify dose of chemotherapy prior to its dispensing initial dose
1.	1.
2.	2.

Page 1 of 2

Date of order: **4-7-10**	Time of order: **1400**

PRE MEDS:

[ ] Dexamethasone ____ mg PO/IV 30 minutes before chemo   *usual range = 4-20 mg*
[ ] Acetaminophen 650 mg PO 30 minutes before chemo
[ ] Diphenhydramine ____mg PO/IV 20 minutes before chemo   *usual range = 12.5-50 mg*
[ ] Ranitidine 150 mg PO 30 minutes before chemo
[✓] Ranitidine 50 mg IV over 15-30 minutes before chemo
[ ] Other_____
[ ] Other_____

Emetogenicity	Minimal	[ ] No antiemetic premedication required
	Low	[ ] Prochlorperazine 10 mg PO X 1
		[✓] Lorazepam **1** mg PO X 1 *usual range 1-2 mg*
	Moderate	[ ] Ondansetron 16 mg PO DAILY 20-30 minutes pre-chemotherapy
		OR
		[ ] Ondansetron 8 mg IV DAILY 20-30 minutes pre-chemotherapy on Days 1 & 8
		PLUS
		[ ] Dexanethasone 20 mg PO/IV X 1 pre-chemotherapy on Days 1 & 8 *usual range 4-20 mg*
		[ ] Lorazepam _____mg PO/IV X 1 pre-chemotherapy *usual range 1-2 mg*
	High-Very High	[ ] Ondansetron 24 mg PO DAILY 20-30 minutes X 1 pre-chemotherapy
		OR
		[ ] Ondansetron 8 mg IV DAILY 20-30 minutes X 1 pre-chemotherapy
		PLUS
		[ ] Dexamethasone _____ mg PO/IV DAILY 20-30 minutes X 1 pre-chemotherapy *usual range 4-20 mg*
		[ ] Lorazepam 1 mg PO X 1 *usual range 1-2 mg*

AS NEEDED:

[ ] Prochlorperazine 10 mg PO/IV Q 4 hours PRN
[ ] Lorazepam 0.5-2 mg PO/IV Q 4 hours PRN
[ ] Diphenhydramine 25-50 mg PO/IV Q 4 hours PRN
[ ] Metoclopramide 10 mg PO/IV Q 6 hours PRN

OTHERS:

[ ] _____
[ ] _____
[ ] _____

[✓] **HYDRATION**   [ ] **HYDRATION NOT REQUIRED**

CHEMOTHERAPY ORDERS

Date of order 7-4	Time of order 1600	Day 1 of this order 1	Patient diagnosis Breast CA
Pt name	Birth date	Cycle #	□ Central Line □ Peripheral Line

Actual Weight 45 kg	Ideal Weight kg	Adjusted Weight kg	Height 145 cm	Body Surface Area 1.46 m²

CHEMOTHERAPY ORDERS: For each drug ordered below, fill in all boxes on the corresponding line or indicate n/a if not applicable.

Chemotherapy Drug	Rec dose	BSA/kg	Dose to be given	ROUTE	RATE	FREQUENCY or day #	# OF DOSES
Cytoxan	40mg/kg		1300 mg	IV	over 30 min	1 of 2	1 of 2

PARAMETER(S)	Instructions (Check all that apply)	
	Call Case Mgr/Provider	HOLD
For absolute neutrophils count less than:	[ ]	[ ]
For platelets less than	[ ]	[ ]
For Mucositis Grade 3 or 4	[ ]	[ ]
For serum creatinine greater than:	[ ]	[ ]
Other:	[ ]	[ ]
Other:	[ ]	[ ]

Prescriber Signature (MD/PA-C/ARNP)	Attending MD Signature (*required prior to order submission*)
2nd Attending MD Signature (*required for non standard dose if documentation not available*)	Pharmacist Review Signature
Two RNs must verify dose of chemotherapy prior to administration of initial dose	Two RPhs must verify dose of chemotherapy prior to its dispensing initial dose
1.	1.
2.	2.

Date of order:	Time of order:

PRE MEDS:

[ ] Dexamethasone ___ mg PO/IV 30 minutes before chemo   *usual range = 4-20 mg*
[ ] Acetaminophen 650 mg PO 30 minutes before chemo
[ ] Diphenhydramine ___mg PO/IV 20 minutes before chemo   *usual range = 12.5-50 mg*
[ ] Ranitidine 150 mg PO 30 minutes before chemo
[ ] Ranitidine 50 mg IV over 15-30 minutes before chemo
[ ] Other_____
[ ] Other_____

Emetogenicity	Minimal	[ ] No antiemetic premedication required
	Low	[ ] Prochlorperazine 10 mg PO X 1
		[ ] Lorazepam ____ mg PO X 1 *usual range 1-2 mg*
	Moderate	[ ] Ondansetron 16 mg PO DAILY 20-30 minutes pre-chemotherapy **OR** [ ] Ondansetron 8 mg IV DAILY 20-30 minutes pre-chemotherapy on Days 1 & 8 **PLUS** [ ] Dexanethasone 20 mg PO/IV X 1 pre-chemotherapy on Days 1 & 8 *usual range 4-20 mg* [ ] Lorazepam _____mg PO/IV X 1 pre-chemotherapy *usual range 1-2 mg*
	High-Very High	[✓] Ondansetron 24 mg PO DAILY 20-30 minutes X 1 pre-chemotherapy **OR** [ ] Ondansetron 8 mg IV DAILY 20-30 minutes X 1 pre-chemotherapy **PLUS** [ ] Dexamethasone _____ mg PO/IV DAILY 20-30 minutes X 1 pre-chemotherapy *usual range 4-20 mg* [✓] Lorazepam 1 mg PO X 1 *usual range 1-2 mg*

AS NEEDED:

[ ] Prochlorperazine 10 mg PO/IV Q 4 hours PRN
[ ] Lorazepam 0.5-2 mg PO/IV Q 4 hours PRN
[ ] Diphenhydramine 25-50 mg PO/IV Q 4 hours PRN
[ ] Metoclopramide 10 mg PO/IV Q 6 hours PRN

OTHERS:

[ ] _____
[ ] _____
[ ] _____

[✓] **HYDRATION**   [ ] **HYDRATION NOT REQUIRED**

Page 2 of 2

CHEMOTHERAPY ORDERS

Date of order	Time of order	Day 1 of this order	Patient diagnosis
4-7-11	0630	1	Breast CA

Pt name	Birth date	Cycle #	☑ Central Line ☐ Peripheral Line
Mary Bosworth	10-15-13		

Actual Weight	Ideal Weight	Adjusted Weight	Height	Body Surface Area
45.5 kg	56.8 kg	kg	145 cm	1.34 m²

CHEMOTHERAPY ORDERS: For each drug ordered below, fill in all boxes on the corresponding line or indicate n/a if not applicable.

Chemotherapy Drug	Rec dose	BSA/kg	Dose to be given	ROUTE	RATE	FREQUENCY or day #	# OF DOSES
Paclitaxel	175 mg/ m²		235 mg	IV	Over 3 hrs	#1	1

PARAMETER(S)	Instructions (Check all that apply)	
	Call Case Mgr/Provider	HOLD
For absolute neutrophils count less than:	[ ]	[ ]
For platelets less than	[ ]	[ ]
For Mucositis Grade 3 or 4	[ ]	[ ]
For serum creatinine greater than:	[ ]	[ ]
Other:	[ ]	[ ]
Other:	[ ]	[ ]

Prescriber Signature (MD/PA-C/ARNP)	Attending MD Signature (*required prior to order submission*)
Dr. Ronald Zimmerman	
2nd Attending MD Signature (*required for non standard dose if documentation not available*)	Pharmacist Review Signature
Two RNs must verify dose of chemotherapy prior to administration of initial dose	Two RPhs must verify dose of chemotherapy prior to its dispensing initial dose
1.	1.
2.	2.

Page 1 of 2

Date of order: 4-7-11	Time of order: 0635

PRE MEDS:

[✓] Dexamethasone __8__ mg PO/IV 30 minutes before chemo   *usual range = 4-20 mg*
[ ] Acetaminophen 650 mg PO 30 minutes before chemo
[ ] Diphenhydramine ___ mg PO/IV 20 minutes before chemo   *usual range = 12.5-50 mg*
[ ] Ranitidine 150 mg PO 30 minutes before chemo
[ ] Ranitidine 50 mg IV over 15-30 minutes before chemo
[ ] Other_____
[ ] Other_____

Emetogenicity	Minimal	[ ] No antiemetic premedication required
	Low	[ ] Prochlorperazine 10 mg PO X 1
		[ ] Lorazepam ___ mg PO X 1 *usual range 1-2 mg*
	Moderate	[ ] Ondansetron 16 mg PO DAILY 20-30 minutes pre-chemotherapy
		OR
		[ ] Ondansetron 8 mg IV DAILY 20-30 minutes pre-chemotherapy on Days 1 & 8
		PLUS
		[ ] Dexanethasone 20 mg PO/IV X 1 pre-chemotherapy on Days 1 & 8 *usual range 4-20 mg*
		[ ] Lorazepam ___ mg PO/IV X 1 pre-chemotherapy *usual range 1-2 mg*
	High-Very High	[ ] Ondansetron 24 mg PO DAILY 20-30 minutes X 1 pre-chemotherapy
		OR
		[ ] Ondansetron 8 mg IV DAILY 20-30 minutes X 1 pre-chemotherapy
		PLUS
		[ ] Dexamethasone ____ mg PO/IV DAILY 20-30 minutes X 1 pre-chemotherapy *usual range 4-20 mg*
		[ ] Lorazepam 1 mg PO X 1 *usual range 1-2 mg*

AS NEEDED:

[ ] Prochlorperazine 10 mg PO/IV Q 4 hours PRN
[ ] Lorazepam 0.5-2 mg PO/IV Q 4 hours PRN
[ ] Diphenhydramine 25-50 mg PO/IV Q 4 hours PRN
[ ] Metoclopramide 10 mg PO/IV Q 6 hours PRN

OTHERS:

[ ] _____
[ ] _____
[ ] _____

[ ] **HYDRATION**   [✓] **HYDRATION NOT REQUIRED**

Page 2 of 2

CHEMOTHERAPY ORDERS

Date of order 6-7-10	Time of order 1245	Day 1 of this order 1 of 4	Patient diagnosis Prostate CA

Pt name *Larry Jones*	Birth date 1-1-01	Cycle #	☐ Central Line ☐ Peripheral Line

Actual Weight 46 kg	Ideal Weight 57 kg	Adjusted Weight kg	Height 145 cm	Body Surface Area 1.34 m²

CHEMOTHERAPY ORDERS: For each drug ordered below, fill in all boxes on the corresponding line or indicate n/a if not applicable.

Chemotherapy Drug	Rec dose	BSA/kg	Dose to be given	ROUTE	RATE	FREQUENCY or day #	# OF DOSES
VP-16	2 x 35 mg/m² per day		100 mg	IV	over 60 min	# 1 of 4	1 of 4

PARAMETER(S)	Instructions (Check all that apply)	
	Call Case Mgr/Provider	HOLD
For absolute neutrophils count less than:	[ ]	[ ]
For platelets less than	[ ]	[ ]
For Mucositis Grade 3 or 4	[ ]	[ ]
For serum creatinine greater than:	[ ]	[ ]
Other:	[ ]	[ ]
Other:	[ ]	[ ]

Prescriber Signature (MD/PA-C/ARNP) *Dr. John Gaffney*	Attending MD Signature (*required prior to order submission*)
2nd Attending MD Signature (*required for non standard dose if documentation not available*)	Pharmacist Review Signature
Two RNs must verify dose of chemotherapy prior to administration of initial dose	Two RPhs must verify dose of chemotherapy prior to its dispensing initial dose
1.	1.
2.	2.

Page 1 of 2

| Date of order: 6-10-10 | Time of order: 1200 |

PRE MEDS:

[ ] Dexamethasone ___ mg PO/IV 30 minutes before chemo   *usual range = 4-20 mg*
[ ] Acetaminophen 650 mg PO 30 minutes before chemo
[✓] Diphenhydramine 12.5 mg PO/IV 20 minutes before chemo   *usual range = 12.5-50 mg*
[ ] Ranitidine 150 mg PO 30 minutes before chemo
[✓] Ranitidine 50 mg IV over 15-30 minutes before chemo
[ ] Other_____
[ ] Other_____

Emetogenicity	Minimal	[ ] No antiemetic premedication required
	Low	[ ] Prochlorperazine 10 mg PO X 1
		[ ] Lorazepam ____ mg PO X 1 *usual range 1-2 mg*
	Moderate	[ ] Ondansetron 16 mg PO DAILY 20-30 minutes pre-chemotherapy
		OR
		[ ] Ondansetron 8 mg IV DAILY 20-30 minutes pre-chemotherapy on Days 1 & 8
		PLUS
		[ ] Dexanethasone 20 mg PO/IV X 1 pre-chemotherapy on Days 1 & 8 *usual range 4-20 mg*
		[ ] Lorazepam _____ mg PO/IV X 1 pre-chemotherapy *usual range 1-2 mg*
	High-Very High	[✓] Ondansetron 24 mg PO DAILY 20-30 minutes X 1 pre-chemotherapy
		OR
		[ ] Ondansetron 8 mg IV DAILY 20-30 minutes X 1 pre-chemotherapy
		PLUS
		[ ] Dexamethasone ____ mg PO/IV DAILY 20-30 minutes X 1 pre-chemotherapy *usual range 4-20 mg*
		[ ] Lorazepam 1 mg PO X 1 *usual range 1-2 mg*

AS NEEDED:

[ ] Prochlorperazine 10 mg PO/IV Q 4 hours PRN
[ ] Lorazepam 0.5-2 mg PO/IV Q 4 hours PRN
[ ] Diphenhydramine 25-50 mg PO/IV Q 4 hours PRN
[ ] Metoclopramide 10 mg PO/IV Q 6 hours PRN

OTHERS:

[ ] _____
[ ] _____
[ ] _____

[ ] HYDRATION   **[✓] HYDRATION NOT REQUIRED**

Page 2 of 2

Total Parenteral Nutrition Orders

Exercise

Process the following total parenteral nutrition (TPN) orders. Once each order is processed, print the medication label, pull the medication from stock, and prepare the medication.

HT: **133** cm   WT: **62** kg

Adult *Total* Parenteral Nutrition Order Form (Central Line Only)

| Date **11-2-10** | Is central line access in place? [ ]No [✓]Yes |
| Time **0730** | Type **grosshong**   Date placed _____ |

Please note: Prescribers must make selections in section 1-6 of form

1. Base Formula (Check one)	2. Infusion Schedule
[ ] Standard Base: dextrose 20% and amino acids (AA) 4.25% (D40W mL and AA 8.5% 500 mL)	Rate: **100** mL/hour_____
[ ] Individual base: Dextrose ___% and AA ___%:	**Cycling Schedule (home TPN only)**
(final concentration)	Cycle____ mL fluid over ____ hours
OR	
Dextrose ___% ___mL	Begin at _____
AA ___% ___mL	

3. Standard Electrolytes/Additives	OR Specify Individualized Electrolytes/Additives	
Check here [ ]	Specify amount of electrolyte	Check all the apply
NaCl 40 mEq / L	NaCl _____ mEq / L	[ ] Adult MVI 10 mLs / day
NaAc 20 mEq / L	NaAc _____ mEq / L	[ ] MTE – 5 3 mLs / day
KCl 20 mEq / L	NaPhos _____ mEq / L	[✓] Regular Human Insulin
Kphos 22 mEq / L	KCl _____ mEq / L	**15** units / Liter
CaGlu 4.7 mEq / L	KAc _____ mEq / L	[ ] Vitamin C 500 mg / day
MagSO4 8 mEq / L	Kphos _____ mEq / L	[✓] 2. antagonis **50** mg / day
Adult MVI 10 mLs / day	CaGlu _____ mEq / L	drug **Zantac**
MTE-5 3 mLs / day	Mag SO4 _____ mEq / L	[ ] Other additives
DO NOT USE IN RENAL DYSFUNCTION!	Maximum Phosphate (Na phos _____	
	40 mEq / L or K phos 44 mEq / L _____	
	and maximum clearance 10 mEq / L	

4. Lipids (Check one)	5. Blood Glucose monitoring orders
Infuse lipids over 12 hours IV	Blood glucose monitoring every **6** hours with
[ ] 20% 250 mL every Tuesday/Thursday	sliding scale regular human insulin.
[✓] 20% 250 mL every day	Route (Circle one) SQ (IV)
[ ] 20% 250 mL every other day	**Sliding Scale** (Check one)
[ ] Other schedule	[ ] Sliding scale per T and T protocol
_____	[ ] Individualized sliding scale (write below)

Additional Orders (All patients)	6. Routine Laboratory Orders (Check all that apply)
1. Consult Nutrition Support Team.	[ ] BMP, Mg, Phos every AM X 3 days then every Monday & Thursday
2. CMP, Mg, Phos, triglyceride, prealbumin in the AM.	[ ] Prealbumin every Monday
3. Weigh patient daily.	[ ] Metabolic study per RT (University only)
4. Strict I/O & document in chart.	[ ] 24 hour UUN and creatinine clearance
5. Keep TPN line inviolate.	
6. If TPN interrupted for any reason, hang D10W@ current TPN rate.	

Physician Signature

HT: **162** cm   WT: **49.5** kg

Adult *Total* Parenteral Nutrition Order Form (Central Line Only)

Date **7-7-10**	Is central line access in place? [ ]No [✓]Yes
Time **2213**	Type **Grosshong** Date placed **3-27-10**

Please note: Prescribers must make selections in section 1-6 of form

1. Base Formula (Check one)	2. Infusion Schedule
[ ] Standard Base: dextrose 20% and amino acids (AA) 4.25% (D40W mL and AA 8.5% 500 mL)	Rate: **83** mL/hour_____
[ ] Individual base: Dextrose **25** % and AA **5** %:	**Cycling Schedule (home TPN only)**
(final concentration)	Cycle_____ mL fluid over _____ hours
OR	Begin at _____
Dextrose____% ____mL	
AA____% ____mL	

3. Standard Electrolytes/Additives	OR Specify Individualized Electrolytes/Additives	
Check here [ ]	Specify amount of electrolyte	Check all the apply
NaCl 40 mEq / L	NaCl **30** mEq / L	[✓]Adult MVI 10 mLs / day _____
NaAc 20 mEq / L	NaAc **20** mEq / L	[✓]MTE – 5 3 mLs / day _____
KCl 20 mEq / L	NaPhos____ mEq / L	[ ] Regular Human Insulin
Kphos 22 mEq / L	KCl **20** mEq / L	____ units / Liter
CaGlu 4.7 mEq / L	KAc____ mEq / L	[ ] Vitamin C 500 mg / day
MagSO4 8 mEq / L	Kphos **20** mEq / L	[✓]H 2 antagonis **50** mg / day
Adult MVI 10 mLs / day	CaGlu____ mEq / L	drug **Zantac**
MTE-5 3 mLs / day	Mag SO4 **10** mEq / L	[ ] Other additives
DO NOT USE IN RENAL DYSFUNCTION!	Maximum Phosphate (Na phos _____	
	40 mEq / L or K phos 44 mEq / L _____	
	and maximum clearance 10 mEq / L	

4. Lipids (Check one)	5. Blood Glucose monitoring orders
Infuse lipids over 12 hours IV	Blood glucose monitoring every **48** hours with
[ ] 20% 250 mL every Tuesday/Thursday	sliding scale regular human insulin.
[✓]20% 250 mL every day	Route (Circle one) (SQ) IV
[ ] 20% 250 mL every other day	**Sliding Scale** (Check one)
[ ] Other schedule	[✓]Sliding scale per T and T protocol
_____	[ ] Individualized sliding scale (write below)

Additional Orders (All patients)	6. Routine Laboratory Orders (Check all that apply)
1. Consult Nutrition Support Team.	[✓]BMP, Mg, Phos every AM X 3 days then every Monday & Thursday
2. CMP, Mg, Phos, triglyceride, prealbumin in the AM.	[ ] Prealbumin every Monday
3. Weigh patient daily.	[ ] Metabolic study per RT (University only)
4. Strict I/O & document in chart.	[✓]24 hour UUN and creatinine clearance
5. Keep TPN line inviolate.	
6. If TPN interrupted for any reason, hang D10W@ current TPN rate.	

Physician Signature

HT: **152** cm   WT: **52** kg

Adult *Total* Parenteral Nutrition Order Form (Central Line Only)

Date **3-3-10**	Is central line access in place? [ ]No [✓]Yes
Time **0645**	Type **Grosshong** Date placed **3-2-10**

Please note: Prescribers must make selections in section 1-6 of form

1. Base Formula (Check one)	2. Infusion Schedule
[✓] Standard Base: dextrose 20% and amino acids (AA) 4.25% (D40W mL and AA 8.5% 500 mL)	Rate: **100** mL/hour_____
[ ] Individual base: Dextrose ___ % and AA ___ %:	**Cycling Schedule (home TPN only)**
(final concentration)	Cycle____ mL fluid over ____ hours
OR	
Dextrose ___ % ___ mL	Begin at _____
AA ___ % ___ mL	

3. Standard Electrolytes/Additives	OR Specify Individualized Electrolytes/Additives	
Check here [✓]	Specify amount of electrolyte	Check all the apply
NaCl 40 mEq / L	NaCl ____ mEq / L	[ ] Adult MVI 10 mLs / day
NaAc 20 mEq / L	NaAc ____ mEq / L	[ ] MTE – 5 3 mLs / day
KCl 20 mEq / L	NaPhos ____ mEq / L	[ ] Regular Human Insulin
Kphos 22 mEq / L	KCl ____ mEq / L	____ units / Liter
CaGlu 4.7 mEq / L	KAc ____ mEq / L	[ ] Vitamin C 500 mg / day
MagSO4 8 mEq / L	Kphos ____ mEq / L	[ ] H 2 antagonis ____ mg / day
Adult MVI 10 mLs / day	CaGlu ____ mEq / L	drug
MTE-5 3 mLs / day	Mag SO4 ____ mEq / L	[ ] Other additives
DO NOT USE IN RENAL DYSFUNCTION!	Maximum Phosphate (Na phos _____ 40 mEq / L or K phos 44 mEq / L _____ and maximum clearance 10 mEq / L	

4. Lipids (Check one)	5. Blood Glucose monitoring orders
Infuse lipids over 12 hours IV	Blood glucose monitoring every ____ hours with
[ ] 20% 250 mL every Tuesday/Thursday	sliding scale regular human insulin.
[✓] 20% 250 mL every day	Route (Circle one) SQ IV
[ ] 20% 250 mL every other day	**Sliding Scale** (Check one)
[ ] Other schedule	[ ] Sliding scale per T and T protocol
_____	[ ] Individualized sliding scale (write below)

Additional Orders (All patients)	6. Routine Laboratory Orders (Check all that apply)
1. Consult Nutrition Support Team.	[✓] BMP, Mg, Phos every AM X 3 days then every Monday & Thursday
2. CMP, Mg, Phos, triglyceride, prealbumin in the AM.	[ ] Prealbumin every Monday
3. Weigh patient daily.	[ ] Metabolic study per RT (University only)
4. Strict I/O & document in chart.	[✓] 24 hour UUN and creatinine clearance
5. Keep TPN line inviolate.	
6. If TPN interrupted for any reason, hang D10W@ current TPN rate.	

Physician Signature